Heal Your Wealth

How Nurses, APRNs, and Healthcare Professionals Break the Paycheck Cycle and Build Generational Wealth

Caroline Oloo, MSN, FNP-BC

APRN CAN DO IT, TOO.

Contents

INTRODUCTION

Nobody Taught Us This

On why the most essential workers in healthcare are also among the most financially unprepared, and what this book does about it

I did not set out to write a financial book. I set out to survive, then to build, and eventually to teach, the book was what grew from all three.

I set out to be a nurse. Then a nurse practitioner. Then a clinical operations executive. Then an entrepreneur building a pharmaceutical distribution company across East Africa. Then a podcast host teaching financial literacy to healthcare professionals who were living the exact financial struggles I had spent years climbing out of. This book grew from all of that, from looking back at the distance I had traveled and realizing that the hardest part of the journey was not clinical. It was financial. And that the map for navigating it simply did not exist in a form that spoke directly to people like me. Each step on that list was a choice made before the next one was visible.

So I wrote it.

> ***The most educated, most essential, most overworked professionals in healthcare are also, consistently, among the most financially unprepared. This is not an accident. It is a gap. And gaps can be closed.***

The Gap This Book Fills

Nursing school teaches you how to save a life. It does not teach you how to build one, not financially. In the years of anatomy and pharmacology and clinical simulation and board preparation, there is almost no instruction on the mechanics of money: how debt compounds, how credit works, what an index fund is, why your employer's 403(b) match is one of the most powerful financial tools available to you and how to use it, what it means to build net worth rather than simply earn income, how to protect everything you build so that a single unprotected event cannot dismantle years of work. It teaches you how to perform under pressure and how to care for others, and it leaves the care of your own financial life entirely to chance.

This gap is not unique to nursing. It extends across the entire healthcare workforce, to physician assistants and pharmacists and therapists and allied health professionals who graduated with significant clinical knowledge, meaningful debt, and almost no financial literacy. They enter careers that pay real salaries and face real financial complexity, equipped with the training to manage a patient's most critical moments and almost no training for managing their own financial ones. It runs through every healthcare profession, and through every family that sent someone into one of them.

The result is predictable, and it is everywhere: brilliant clinicians living paycheck to paycheck. Healthcare professionals working seven days a week not because they want to but because the budget requires it. Nurses in the overtime trap, performing financial wellness for their colleagues while privately counting down to the next deposit. First-generation professionals sending money home to family abroad while their own savings accounts hold less than one month of expenses. People who sacrificed enormously to build a clinical career, and who deserve so much better from the financial life that career makes possible. Brilliant clinicians living paycheck to paycheck is not a coincidence, it is a systemic outcome.

This book is for all of them. For all of you. It is the book that should have existed before the first paycheck arrived.

Who I Am and Why This Is My Story to Tell

I was born and raised in Kenya. I came to the United States as an information technology professional and pivoted to nursing, not a small pivot, and not one made without cost. My sister Collet funded my nursing education. My father, Mr. Jacob, believed in education with the fervor of someone who understood, intuitively, that knowledge was the asset that could not be taken from you. He lived paycheck to paycheck his entire life, not from lack of ambition, but from lack of financial information. I watched that pattern. I absorbed it. And then, after years of living a version of it myself in America, the two jobs, the credit card debt, the overtime that produced income that somehow disappeared before the next cycle, I decided to understand it well enough to break it. That origin is not incidental; it is the lens through which everything in this book was learned.

Today I am a board-certified Family Nurse Practitioner managing clinical teams across four states. I am Director of Clinical Operations. I am the co-founder of Icon Oncology Supply, a pharmaceutical distribution company operating in Kenya and expanding across East Africa. I wrote From Bedside to Boardroom: A Nurse's Roadmap to Executive Leadership. None of those roles were visible to me when I started, they became possible because I refused to accept the first option as the ceiling.

And I am, at my core, the nurse who sat at a kitchen table with every financial statement laid out in front of her and decided that the paycheck-to-paycheck life she had inherited was not the life she would pass forward. That kitchen table is where this book began, and it is where every reader of this book is invited to begin as well.

That decision is the origin of this book.

How to Use This Book

Heal Your Wealth is organized as a journey, eleven chapters that move from financial awareness through debt elimination, budgeting, investing, real estate, entrepreneurship, identity, protection, and legacy. Each chapter opens with a moment from clinical life, moves into principle and strategy grounded in the particular realities of healthcare work, and closes with a Boardroom Moment: reflection questions and concrete action steps designed to move ideas from the page into your actual financial life. The journey is sequential by design, each chapter builds on the one before it, which is how financial transformation actually works.

You can read it from beginning to end, and I recommend that you do, at least once, because the chapters build on each other in ways that reward the sequence. You can also return to specific chapters as your financial situation evolves: Chapter 3 when the debt feels overwhelming, Chapter 6 when you are ready to begin investing, Chapter 10 when you have built enough to need to protect it, Chapter 11 when you are ready to think about what you are leaving behind. The book is built to meet you wherever you are, and to stay useful as your situation changes.

The book does not assume a specific income level, a specific debt load, or a specific starting point. It assumes only that you are a healthcare professional who is ready to take your financial life as seriously as you take your clinical one, and that you are willing to be honest about where you are in order to get somewhere different. It assumes only that you are ready, and readiness, it turns out, is the only prerequisite.

A Note on Impostor Syndrome

Before you begin, I want to address something that may be sitting quietly in the background as you hold this book: the feeling that financial literacy is for someone else. That wealth-building is for people who started with more, earned more, knew more from the beginning. That the nurses and APRNs and allied health professionals who have built real financial freedom are somehow different from you in ways that make their outcomes unavailable to your life. That feeling is not evidence of limitation, it is evidence of a gap in what you were given, not what you are capable of.

They are not different. I am not different. The clinical credential, the immigrant background, the first-generation professional journey, the family obligations spanning two continents, the debt, the overtime trap, the kitchen table moment with every statement in front of me, none of that is a story of exceptional advantage. It is a story of a decision, made in the middle of an ordinary life, to do something different with the financial reality that decision created. The outcomes differ because the decisions differed, and decisions can be changed starting today.

You can make that decision. You already have, in some sense, you picked up this book. Now let us make it mean something.

> ***Financial freedom is not reserved for people who started in a different place than you did. It is built by people who decided, at whatever point in their journey that decision became possible, to stop waiting and start building.***

The Promise of This Book

By the time you close the final chapter, you will have a net worth calculation for the first time, or an updated one that you understand. You will have a debt elimination plan with a sequence and a target. You will have a budget built around your baseline income that does not require overtime to function. You will understand your employer's retirement benefits, in enough detail to maximize them, and you will have a starting framework for investing that does not require a finance degree to execute. You will understand what real estate can do for a healthcare professional's financial life and how to approach it practically. You will have confronted the financial identity you inherited, named the beliefs that have been governing your decisions without your permission, and chosen a different story. You will also have something harder to quantify and more important than any number: a different relationship with money.

And you will have, in the final chapter, a legacy statement, a declaration of what you are building, why you are building it, and who it is ultimately for.

That is the promise. Not that the work will be easy. Not that the path will be without difficulty or setback or the occasional month that does not go as planned. But that the map exists. That it was written by someone who has walked the terrain. And that every step it describes is available to you, beginning with the next one. Not that the journey will be easy, that it is possible, that the map exists, and that every step is available to you.

Before You Turn the Page

Write down your current financial reality in one sentence. Not the comfortable version. The true one. The distance between those two sentences is the work, and this book was built to take you the full distance.

Write down what you want your financial life to look like in ten years. Be specific.

Keep both sentences. We will return to them in Chapter 11.

The distance between those two sentences is the journey this book is designed to take you on.

Nobody taught us this. We are teaching it now, and teaching it to everyone who comes after us.

We are teaching it now.

Caroline Oloo, MSN, FNP-BC

PhD Candidate | Director of Clinical Operations | Entrepreneur

Begin with Chapter 1: The Paycheck That Changed Everything

CHAPTER ONE

The Paycheck That Changed Everything

On earning your first real income, and discovering that money is only half the equation

I remember the exact moment I saw the number. That moment marked the beginning of a journey I had not yet been taught to take.

It was a direct deposit notification on my phone, my first paycheck as a registered nurse. I stared at it the way you stare at something you have wanted for so long that when it finally arrives, you almost cannot believe it is real. This was not a student stipend. This was not a part-time shift at a clinic making ends meet. This was a nurse's salary. My nurse's salary. Earned through years of sacrifice, late nights studying pharmacology, clinical rotations that tested every limit I had, and a leap of faith that had cost my sister Collet more than I could ever fully repay. Nothing in nursing school had prepared me for what came next.

I sat down. I cried. And then I started planning. The planning felt like power, until I realized I did not know what to plan for.

> ***I had worked so hard to earn money. What nobody had taught me was what to do with it. Earning and building are two very different skills, and only one of them is taught.***

The Dream of Living Alone

For as long as I could remember, living independently had been the symbol of everything I was working toward. Not just in a practical sense, a roof, a key, a space of my own, but in a deeper sense. It meant I had made it. It meant the investment my family had made in me had returned something real. It meant Collet could finally exhale. Independence was the goal, but I had no map for how to fund it wisely.

My sister had done more than support my nursing education. She had carried me. She had funded tuition when I had nothing, believed in my pivot from IT to nursing when the path was unclear, and never once made me feel like a burden, even when I surely was one. When that paycheck landed, I thought about her first. The sense of pride I felt was wrapped up entirely in what I imagined she would feel: relief. Fulfillment. The quiet satisfaction of watching someone you love finally stand on their own. The debt I carried to her was never financial, it was gratitude I could only repay by succeeding.

For Collet

The woman who funded a dream she never doubted.

This chapter, and this book, exists because of your sacrifice.

You gave me the foundation. What I built on it is my gift back to you.

I was going to get my own apartment. I was going to furnish it beautifully. I was going to build the life I had imagined through every exhausting shift, every board exam, every moment of doubt. I had a plan. I had a spreadsheet. I had ambition and energy and a brand-new paycheck. I had a vision for the life, but not yet the financial literacy to build it.

What I did not have was financial literacy. That gap would cost me more than any bill I ever received.

The Education No One Gave Us

Here is what nursing school teaches you: pathophysiology, pharmacology, clinical assessment, patient advocacy, evidence-based practice. Here is what nursing school does not teach you: how money works. How debt compounds. How a credit card with a twenty-three percent interest rate quietly dismantles the financial foundation you are trying to build. How the apartment you qualify for on paper can cost you far more than the rent line suggests once you add utilities, parking, renter's insurance, and the slow drain of a lifestyle you are not yet equipped to afford. Everything on that list made me a better clinician, and nothing on it made me a better steward of money.

I was not financially ignorant from carelessness. I was financially ignorant because no one had ever taught me. And I am not alone. Across the healthcare profession, in hospitals, clinics, and nursing units on every continent, brilliant, dedicated clinicians are earning respectable salaries and still living paycheck to paycheck. Not because of laziness. Because of a gap in our formation that the system never addressed and the curriculum never covered. Ignorance is not a character flaw, it is an information gap, and information gaps can be closed.

> ***You can pass every board exam and still fail the most important financial test of your career, because no one ever put it on the syllabus.***

The Credit Card and the Beautiful Apartment

My first financial move after that paycheck was to apply for credit cards. I made that move not out of recklessness, but out of a system I did not yet understand.

I want to be honest with you about this, because honesty is the only thing that makes a book like this worth reading. I did not apply for credit cards because I was reckless. I applied because I needed to furnish my apartment, and I had been told, in various ways, that credit was how adults managed large purchases. What I had not been told was the difference between using credit as a tool and using it as a substitute for money I did not yet have.

I found a beautiful apartment. It was in a neighborhood I loved, at a price point that felt just within reach, which, as I would soon discover, is not the same thing as actually being within reach. I signed the lease with confidence. I moved in. I bought furniture on credit. I bought kitchen appliances on credit. I bought scrubs and shoes and the small, satisfying objects that make a new space feel like home. And for a brief, extraordinary moment, everything felt exactly right. It looked like the life I had worked for, and it cost more than I had planned to pay for it.

Then the bills arrived.

The First Month Reality Check

Rent:	Large portion of take-home pay
Utilities + internet:	Surprise, higher than estimated
Credit card minimum:	Growing faster than expected
Groceries:	Forgot to budget for these
Scrubs, shoes, work supplies:	Not optional expenses
Savings:	$0

The math did not lie. The math never lies. I just had not done it honestly.

The question I found myself asking at the end of that first month was one that millions of nurses ask in silence, too embarrassed to say it out loud: do I eat, pay bills, or go shopping for the scrubs I need for work? It sounds like an exaggeration. It was not. It was the precise, humbling arithmetic of someone who had finally earned a real income and had no idea how to govern it. That question is not unique to me, it is the silent math of nurses across every shift, every unit, every continent.

The Overtime Trap, My Personal Introduction

There is a solution that seems obvious when you are staring at a shortfall: work more. Pick up an extra shift. Take a second job. Earn your way out of the gap. Working more feels like the answer right up until the moment you realize it is not.

I did exactly that. After my standard three twelve-hour shifts, already among the most physically and emotionally demanding workdays any profession produces, I added more. I worked shifts at a second hospital. I came home exhausted in ways that went deeper than tired. I slept on days off not because I wanted to but because my body had no other option. And I watched my bank account improve, briefly, before the cycle reasserted itself with quiet efficiency. More hours meant more exhaustion, and exhaustion, it turns out, is its own kind of expensive.

More income meant more spending. Not because I was undisciplined, though I will not pretend discipline was never a factor, but because exhaustion is expensive. When you are too tired to cook, you order food. When you are too depleted to make thoughtful decisions, you buy convenience. When your only reward for an unbearable week is a small pleasure, you take it. The relief of the purchase outlasts the regret, at least for a few hours. The pattern repeats itself with the quiet efficiency of a system that was never designed to stop.

This is not a moral failing. This is human neuroscience applied to structural exhaustion. And it is one of the most common financial patterns in nursing, precisely because our work is so demanding that the spending becomes a coping mechanism rather than a choice. It is structural, and understanding the structure is the first step to escaping it.

> ***I was not spending my way into debt. I was recovering from work in the only ways I knew how, and recovery, it turns out, is not free.***

The cycle I entered in those first years as an RN is one I have watched repeat itself in nurses across two continents, in hospitals from Texas to Nairobi, in colleagues who are brilliant and hardworking and genuinely confused about why the math never seems to add up. Work. Earn. Spend. Owe. Work more. The hamster wheel does not slow down because you run faster. It speeds up. I watched that cycle spin with increasing speed before I finally understood how to step off it.

What Paycheck to Paycheck Actually Feels Like

I want to describe this plainly, because the phrase 'living paycheck to paycheck' has become so common that it has lost its texture. Giving the feeling a name is the first act of taking it seriously.

It feels like this: you check your bank balance before every purchase over twenty dollars. You decline social invitations not because you do not want to go, but because you cannot do the math on the dinner. You know, within forty-eight hours, when your next deposit will hit, not because you are organized, but because you are counting on it to cover something already overdue. You avoid opening certain bills. You feel a steady, low-grade anxiety that does not announce itself loudly but never fully leaves, the financial equivalent of a headache you have grown so accustomed to that you have stopped calling it a headache and started calling it normal. That headache does not go away on its own, it requires a deliberate decision to treat it.

It is not normal. It is a symptom. And like every symptom a good clinician encounters, it is information. It is telling you something about the system, not about your worth, not about your intelligence, not about your future. About the system. And systems can be changed. Symptoms point to causes, and causes, once identified, can be addressed.

The Belief Underneath the Behavior

Here is what I have come to understand, after years of living through this pattern and then learning my way out of it: the spending was never the real problem. The belief was. The behavior was always downstream of the belief, and beliefs are the one thing we can actually change.

I believed, at some level I had never consciously examined, that money was something that happened to you, that arrived, that circulated, that left, rather than something you directed. I believed that earning more would automatically mean having more, because no one had ever shown me the mechanism between the two. I believed that financial struggle was a temporary condition I would outgrow once I reached the next salary level, the next job, the next promotion. I was always one step away from the version of financial life where things finally made sense. Unexamined beliefs govern more financial decisions than any budget ever written.

That step never came, not because the promotions did not, but because the belief had not changed. And until the belief changes, the behavior follows the same arc regardless of the income level. I have watched this truth play out in nurses earning forty thousand dollars a year and nurses earning four hundred thousand. The number on the paycheck is not the variable that matters most. The story you tell yourself about money is.

> ***You do not have a money problem. You have a money belief problem. And beliefs, unlike bank balances, you can change starting today.***

This is the work of this book. Not budgeting for its own sake. Not investing as a performance of responsibility. The real work, the work that precedes all the practical strategies in the chapters ahead, is identifying the belief that has been governing your financial life without your permission, and replacing it with something that actually serves you. It is not easy work, but it is the most important work a healthcare professional can do for her financial future.

My belief, unexamined, was: money is for surviving. The belief I chose, once I finally chose it: money is for building. The new belief did not arrive all at once, it was built, one deliberate decision at a time.

That single shift in thinking changed everything that followed. It can change everything for you too.

A Note to the Nurse Reading This at 2 a.m.

If you picked up this book during a break between shifts, or after a long day when the bank notification did not say what you hoped, or because someone handed it to you and said this might help, I want you to know something before we go any further. Wherever you are starting from, the starting point is not the end of the story.

What you are carrying is not a character flaw. The financial anxiety, the debt, the second job, the sense that everyone else has figured out something you haven't, none of it is evidence of a deficiency in you. It is evidence of a gap in what you were taught. A gap that exists because the systems that trained you needed your clinical skills far more urgently than they cared about your retirement account. It is evidence of a gap in what you were given, and gaps can be filled.

You are not broken. You are not behind. You are simply at the beginning of a different kind of education, one that this book is designed to give you.

And wherever you are starting from, whatever the balance, whatever the debt, whatever the story, you are exactly on time.

BOARDROOM MOMENT

Heal Your Wealth, Chapter 1 Reflection

Set aside fifteen minutes, find a quiet space, and answer these questions honestly. There are no wrong answers, only true ones.

1. Think back to your first significant paycheck, as a nurse, as a clinician, or in any role that felt like arrival. What did you do with it? What were you feeling? What did you believe, in that moment, that money would mean for your life?
2. What is one money belief you inherited from your family or your upbringing that you have never consciously examined? Write it down exactly as you would say it to yourself. Then ask: is this belief true? Is it serving me?
3. If you are currently in a paycheck-to-paycheck cycle, or have been in the past, what emotion does that cycle produce most often? Shame? Anxiety? Resignation? Naming the emotion is the first step to separating it from your identity.
4. What would your financial life look like in five years if the only thing that changed was your belief about what money is for? Write that version of your life in one paragraph. Save it. We will return to it at the end of this book.

Write your answers down. The act of writing is the beginning of your wealth shift.

* * *

In Chapter 2, we do the work that most financial books skip: we build your honest financial baseline. Not the version you wish were true. The version that actually is. Because the only way to build something real is to start from where you actually are, not where you hoped you would be by now.

The good news is this: knowing your number, however uncomfortable, is the first act of financial courage. And courage, as every nurse already knows, is not the absence of fear. It is moving forward anyway.

Continue to Chapter 2: Know Your Number

CHAPTER TWO

Know Your Number

On facing the truth about where you stand, and why that courage is the beginning of everything

There is a moment, somewhere in the middle of the overtime trap, when the exhaustion becomes clarifying. That moment of clarity is the beginning of financial intentionality, and it costs nothing except honesty.

Not immediately. First it just hurts. You work more hours than your body was designed to sustain, you watch your bank account improve and then contract, you tell yourself next month will be different, and then next month arrives and looks exactly like the one before it. The cycle is so consistent, so predictable, that it starts to feel like weather, something that happens to you rather than something you are participating in. The cycle is painful before it becomes informative, and most people stop at the pain.

But then, if you are paying attention, something shifts. The exhaustion stops being a complaint and becomes a question. You stop asking why is this so hard and start asking what am I actually doing with everything I am working this hard for? That question, that precise, uncomfortable, honest question, was the beginning of my financial education.

I had been a registered nurse for a couple of years. I had two jobs, a beautiful apartment I could barely afford, a credit card balance that was quietly growing, and a bone-deep tiredness that no amount of sleep seemed to fully address. And one day, almost by accident, I sat down and looked, really looked, at the numbers. Looking back at those numbers was one of the hardest and most necessary things I had ever done.

What I saw changed everything. Truth has a way of doing that, especially when you have been avoiding it.

> ***You cannot fix what you refuse to face. And you cannot build what you have never measured.***

The Woman Who Taught Me What Intentional Looks Like

Before I could become intentional with money, I had to see what intentional looked like up close. I found that model in the most unexpected place: my own sister's living room. Intentionality, I learned, is not a personality trait, it is a practice, and it can be learned.

Collet had always been the steady one. While I was navigating the overwhelm of a new country, a new career, and a lifestyle that was outpacing my income, she was quietly doing something I had not fully registered: building. She owned two properties. One was the home where we lived together, a roof she had provided while I found my footing. The other was an investment property, a second home generating rental income that arrived every month regardless of whether she had worked a single extra shift. Her steadiness was not luck, it was a set of decisions made quietly and consistently over time.

She was not earning significantly more than I was. She was not working seven days a week. She was calculated. She had sat down with her finances, looked at what she had, made a plan that her income could support, and executed it with a discipline that I had admired without ever fully understanding. She did not talk about money constantly. She did not lecture. But watching her, the way she moved through financial decisions with a quiet deliberateness that I had no vocabulary for at the time, planted something in me that was about to take root. That fact stopped me cold the first time I fully registered it.

What Collet Modeled Without Saying a Word

You do not need to earn more to build more. You need to think differently.

A second income stream from an asset is not the same as a second job.

Financial peace is not luck. It is the compounded result of intentional decisions made consistently over time.

Watching someone live this truth is more powerful than any textbook.

I sat with that observation for a long time. My sister was not immune to financial pressure. She was also helping back home in Kenya, contributing to school fees, carrying family responsibility across an ocean, doing what so many immigrant professionals do without it ever appearing on a balance sheet. But she had structured her financial life so that the income was not entirely dependent on her trading more hours for more dollars. She had built something that worked for her even when she was not working. The observation stayed with me because it dismantled the story I had been telling myself about why I was behind.

I wanted that kind of life. I did not yet know how to build it. But for the first time, I had a living example that it was possible, and that it began not with earning more, but with knowing your number. Not knowing how to build something is not a reason to stop, it is a reason to start learning.

The Weight of Two Worlds

I need to pause here and speak to something that does not appear in most personal finance books, because most personal finance books are not written by immigrant nurses who are simultaneously building a life in America and holding up a family in Kenya. This is the chapter of this book that most personal finance books skip entirely.

When I talk about financial pressure, I am not talking only about rent and credit card debt. I am talking about school fees for a younger brother back home. I am talking about the invisible line item in every budget that never gets named but is always accounted for: the responsibility you carry for people who are counting on you from thousands of miles away. The obligation that does not come with a billing statement but arrives as a phone call, a need, a family member who has no one else. The pressure of holding up two worlds while building your own is a weight that has no line item in a standard budget.

This is the financial reality of a large part of the nursing workforce, particularly nurses who have immigrated, who are first-generation professionals, who come from cultures where family financial support is not optional but assumed. You are not just managing your own life. You are managing the downstream effects of your success on everyone who believed in you enough to watch you go.

I took over my brother's school fees. It was not a complicated decision, he needed support, I was the one positioned to provide it, and that is simply how our family operates. But it was another weight on a budget that was already straining. And it clarified something important: I could not afford to stay in the overtime trap. Not financially, and not humanly. I was working to sustain too many things, and I was doing it inefficiently. Something had to change. That decision did not feel like a burden, it felt like what family does, which is exactly why it needed to be planned for.

> ***The financial pressure of carrying two worlds, one in America, one back home, is real, valid, and almost never discussed. It does not make building wealth impossible. It makes intentionality non-negotiable.***

The Decision to Get Intentional

Intentionality sounds like a self-help word. Soft. Abstract. Easy to nod at and harder to actually practice. But for me, in that season of my life, getting intentional meant something concrete and uncomfortable: I sat down with my finances and I did not look away. But in practice, intentionality is nothing more than deciding before the money arrives where it is going.

I wrote down every number. Income from both jobs. Rent. Credit card balances and minimum payments and interest rates. Utilities. Groceries, the actual amount I spent, not the amount I told myself I spent. The money going to Kenya. The incidental expenses that had no category but somehow always appeared. I put it all on paper, in one place, at the same time. The act of writing it down changed it from a vague weight to a specific, solvable problem.

What I saw was clarifying in the way that cold water is clarifying, sudden, sharp, and impossible to mistake for anything other than what it is. I was not building. I was cycling. The two jobs were not creating financial progress. They were funding a lifestyle that had expanded to absorb every additional dollar I brought in, plus some I had borrowed. My net worth, a concept I had not fully understood before that moment, was negative. I owed more than I owned. Cold water wakes you up, it does not hurt you, even when it shocks you.

That number was not shameful. It was information. And information, for someone trained to diagnose and treat, is not a reason for despair. It is a starting point. Shame keeps you stuck; information moves you forward.

What 'Knowing Your Number' Actually Means

NET WORTH = What You Own (Assets) minus What You Owe (Liabilities)

Assets include: savings, investments, property value, retirement accounts, anything of value you could liquidate

Liabilities include: credit card balances, student loans, car loans, medical debt, any money you owe to anyone

If the number is negative: you are in debt. This is your starting line, not your verdict.

If the number is positive: you have a foundation. Now we build on it.

If you have never calculated it: that changes today.

The Downgrade That Was Actually an Upgrade

One of the first intentional decisions I made was the one that felt the most like defeat at the time: I moved to a smaller, less expensive apartment. The smaller apartment felt like failure at the time and functions in memory as one of the best choices I ever made.

I want to sit with that for a moment, because the emotional reality of that decision matters. My beautiful apartment had been a symbol, of arrival, of independence, of the life I had imagined when I was studying for boards at midnight. Leaving it felt like admitting I had been wrong. Like scaling back the dream. Decisions that feel like retreat in the moment are often the ones that look like strategy in hindsight.

It was the opposite. Downgrading my apartment was the first truly strategic financial decision I had made since becoming a nurse. The money I freed from rent did not disappear into the same cycle. For the first time, I was directing it. Toward the credit card balances. Toward building a small emergency fund, a concept I had read about but never actually implemented. Toward the clarity of knowing that what I was paying each month was genuinely sustainable. For the first time, I was directing money rather than watching it leave.

The apartment was smaller. My financial life grew larger. That is a trade I would make again without hesitation.

> ***Downgrading is not retreat. It is strategy. Every great builder knows the difference between what looks like progress and what actually is.***

The Tuition Benefit I Almost Did Not Use

Around this time, something else became available to me that I had not fully investigated: my hospital's tuition assistance program. Benefits are compensation, and compensation left unclaimed is compensation lost.

Many hospitals and healthcare systems offer education benefits, tuition reimbursement, upfront payment plans, or interest-free loans for employees pursuing advanced degrees. These programs exist because hospitals want to retain skilled staff, and supporting education is one of the ways they do it. But in my experience, a significant number of nurses do not fully understand what their employer offers, or they assume the process is too complicated to be worth pursuing. The process is rarely as complicated as it sounds, and the return is almost always worth the paperwork.

My hospital would advance tuition at the start of each semester and reimburse the balance at semester's end, a bridge that made returning to school financially viable in a way it would not otherwise have been. That benefit, combined with a more disciplined approach to my own spending, made the NP program possible. Not easy. Possible. And possible was enough. That benefit changed the trajectory of my career, and it was available to me the entire time I worked there.

I want to be direct here: going back to school while working was one of the hardest things I have done. The hours were brutal. The intellectual load was significant. There were nights when I questioned every decision that had led me to that desk at that hour, studying pharmacology for an advanced exam after a twelve-hour shift. But I had a number in my mind, not just a salary number, but a net worth number, a freedom number, and that number was worth the sacrifice. Hard and worth it are not mutually exclusive, in fact, they almost always travel together.

Benefits Most Nurses Leave on the Table

Tuition reimbursement or advancement, check your hospital's HR portal

403(b) or 401(k) matching, free money that stops the moment you stop contributing

Loan forgiveness programs, Public Service Loan Forgiveness (PSLF) for nonprofit hospital employees

CEU and certification reimbursement, continuing education without out-of-pocket cost

Employee assistance programs, sometimes include financial counseling

Rule of thumb: if your employer offers it and you are not using it, you are leaving compensation on the table.

The Nurses Who Are Still There

I need to tell you about the nurses I know, colleagues, friends, people I have worked alongside in hospitals across multiple states, who are still in the overtime trap today. Not because they are less capable than I am. Not because they have made worse decisions. But because no one ever gave them what I am trying to give you in this book: a framework, a permission structure, and the specific vocabulary to understand what is happening to their money and why.

I know nurses who have worked seven days a week for years, not because they want to, but because the arithmetic of their lives leaves them no other option. The student loans are real. The family obligations are real. The cost of living in the cities where hospitals are concentrated is real. The overtime is not a lifestyle choice. It is a survival strategy that has become a permanent condition because no one ever offered an alternative. The overtime is not a lifestyle choice for them, it is a structural trap that was never designed to have an exit.

This is why financial literacy in nursing education matters so deeply to me. If we taught nurses what I learned the hard way, before they signed their first lease, before they applied for their first credit card, before they picked up their first extra shift in a panic about bills, the trajectory of this profession would shift. Not immediately, and not for everyone, but meaningfully. Enough to matter. A curriculum that creates financially literate graduates would change the profession more than any wage increase.

> ***If financial literacy were part of nursing curriculum, we would graduate clinicians who are not just excellent at saving lives, but equipped to build one.***

What We Learned Growing Up, and What We Have to Unlearn

I grew up in Kenya watching my father live paycheck to paycheck. I watched every adult in my family navigate money the same way, not because they were careless or unambitious, but because that was the only model available. Money arrived. Money was spent on necessities. Whatever remained was small and unreliable. And then it started over. He worked hard his entire life, the problem was never effort, it was information.

Financial literacy was not a kitchen table conversation in my home. It was not a school subject. It was not something the adults around me had been taught, and so they could not teach it to me. This is not a criticism, it is a description of a reality that millions of families share across every continent, every culture, every income level. The cycle of financial struggle persists across generations not because families lack intelligence or work ethic, but because no one breaks the information gap. It was not there because no one had given it to the people sitting at that table, and they could not give what they did not have.

I refuse to accept it as normal. I refused then, in that smaller apartment with my credit card statements laid out in front of me, and I refuse now. Not out of judgment for the people who lived that way before me, I carry nothing but love and gratitude for them, but out of a clear-eyed commitment to being the generation that does it differently. The one who figures it out. The one who writes it down. The one who hands the map to everyone who comes after. Normal is just what we have grown accustomed to, it is not what we are limited to.

That is what this book is. A map. Drawn from the inside of the experience, by someone who got lost in exactly the same places you might be lost in right now.

To Every Nurse Still in the Cycle

You are not behind. You are not broken. You are not proof that wealth is not possible for someone like you. You are exactly where you need to be to make a different decision, which is all that is required to start.

You are in the middle of a story that has not finished yet.

The chapter you are in right now is called Know Your Number.

Turn the page.

The Dream That Became a Direction

Something happened when I started getting honest about my finances: the dream changed shape. Not smaller, bigger. But more specific. Less about a beautiful apartment or a certain lifestyle and more about something I started calling the freedom number. Honesty about money, it turns out, does not make the situation worse, it makes it clearer.

The freedom number is not a salary figure. It is not a retirement account balance. It is the number at which your money works hard enough that you do not have to. The number at which the choice to work an extra shift is genuinely a choice, not a necessity. The number at which the school fees and the family obligations and the student loans and the retirement contributions are all covered, and there is still something left over to direct toward the life you actually want. It is the number at which your money begins to work for you instead of the other way around.

That number looked enormous to me in those early years. It still looked enormous when I was in the NP program, studying nights and weekends while working full time. But it had stopped feeling impossible, because for the first time I had a baseline. I knew where I was starting from. And knowing your starting point, however humbling, is the only way to plot a direction toward where you want to go. Enormous and impossible are different things, and knowing the number made the distance feel crossable.

The dream of becoming a nurse practitioner was not just about the credential or the scope of practice. It was about the freedom number. About building a clinical expertise that could generate income in multiple ways, through practice, through leadership, through entrepreneurship, rather than being permanently dependent on how many hours I could trade in a single week. The credential was the vehicle, the freedom number was the destination.

That dream started with a number on a piece of paper in a smaller apartment. Not with the apartment I wished I had. With the truth of the one I could actually afford. Every transformation starts somewhere specific, mine started there.

> ***The path to financial freedom does not begin with a big salary. It begins with the courage to look honestly at the one you have.***

Your Turn: Build Your Baseline

Below is the framework I wish someone had handed me on the day I finally sat down with my finances. Fill it in with your real numbers, not approximations, not what you hope is true, but the actual figures. This is a private document. No one is grading you. The only purpose it serves is giving you the starting point that changes everything.

ASSETS	Your Estimated Value
Checking account balance	$
Savings account balance	$
Retirement account (401k/403b/IRA)	$
Investment accounts	$
Property value (if you own)	$
Vehicle value (current market)	$
Other assets of value	$
TOTAL ASSETS	$

LIABILITIES	Amount Owed
Student loans (total balance)	$
Credit card balances (all cards)	$
Car loan remaining balance	$
Medical debt	$
Personal loans	$

Any other debt	$
TOTAL LIABILITIES	$

NET WORTH CALCULATION	
Total Assets	$
Minus Total Liabilities	- $
YOUR NET WORTH	= $

Whatever that number is, positive, negative, or zero, it is the most important financial number you have written down all year. Keep it. We will return to it. Because one of the most powerful things you can do for your financial life is track how this number grows over time. Not obsessively. But consistently. Because a rising net worth is the proof that the strategy is working, and there is nothing more motivating than watching the number you once were afraid to look at begin, slowly and then all at once, to move in your favor.

BOARDROOM MOMENT

Heal Your Wealth, Chapter 2 Reflection

This is your financial baseline exercise. It will take honesty and perhaps twenty minutes. Do not skip it. The discomfort you feel completing it is the discomfort of someone finally telling themselves the truth, and that is exactly where healing begins.

5. Complete the net worth worksheet above using your actual numbers. If you do not have all the figures immediately, gather them before moving to Chapter 3. This is the assignment. Do not proceed without it.
6. Look at your total liabilities. Which single debt, if eliminated, would change how you feel about your finances most significantly? That debt, not necessarily the largest, but the most emotionally heavy, is your first target.
7. Are there benefits your employer offers that you are not currently using? This week, pull up your HR portal or benefits summary and read it in full. Write down one benefit you will act on before the end of the month.
8. Who in your life models financial intentionality the way Collet modeled it for me? If no one comes to mind, that is important information, and it is part of why this book exists. Who could you learn from, formally or informally, starting now?
9. Write one sentence that describes the financial life you are building toward, not the salary, not the title, but the feeling. The freedom. The specific thing that working this hard is ultimately for.

Your number is not your verdict. It is your starting point. And every great journey begins with knowing exactly where you stand.

* * *

In Chapter 3, we address the weight that sits on top of every financial plan a nurse tries to build: debt. Student loans, credit card balances, the specific trap of borrowing to get through a training that the system told you was necessary. We will name it clearly, without shame, and then we will build a strategy for moving through it, not around it, but directly through it.

Because debt is not a life sentence. It is a chapter. And chapters, as you are learning, have endings.

Continue to Chapter 3: The Debt Detox

CHAPTER THREE

The Debt Detox

Accept your reality. Confront it with every tool available to you. Then build your way out.

Nobody talks about debt the way a clinician understands disease.

In nursing, we are trained to do something that most people spend their lives avoiding: look directly at the problem. We do not turn away from a wound because it is uncomfortable. We do not pretend a symptom is not there because naming it feels frightening. We assess, we document, we diagnose, and then we treat — with every tool available, without apology, toward healing.

Financial debt is a wound millions of nurses carry in silence. Not because they are irresponsible, not because they are unintelligent, but because no one ever handed them the clinical equivalent of a treatment protocol. They were given the diagnosis — the balance statement, the interest rate, the minimum payment — but never the plan.

This chapter is the plan.

> ***You treated the most complex patients in your unit without flinching. Your debt deserves the same clinical precision — and the same confidence that healing is possible.***

Accept Your Reality

The first instruction in this chapter is the hardest: accept your reality.

Not the version of your finances you have been telling yourself. Not the approximate figure you carry in your head. Not the number you plan to deal with after the next pay raise, the next tax return, the next promotion. The actual number. The one that lives on the statements you have been opening less frequently than you should.

Acceptance — true acceptance — is not passive. It is not resignation. It is the deliberate act of seeing clearly so that you can move purposefully. In clinical terms, it is the assessment phase: before you can treat anything, you must know exactly what you are treating. Skipping assessment to jump straight to intervention is how nurses make mistakes. And it is how people in debt stay in debt — cycling through half-measures because they never fully confronted the magnitude of what they were dealing with.

I know how uncomfortable this is because I lived it. The moment I spread every statement on my kitchen table — credit cards, student loans, the balance I owed a family member, the store card I had nearly forgotten — was one of the most difficult evenings of my adult life. Not because the numbers were catastrophic. But seeing them all at once, in one place, made it impossible to continue pretending the situation was manageable on its own.

It was not managing itself. And the first step to changing that was admitting it.

The Courage of Acceptance

Accepting your financial reality is not a surrender.
It is the bravest thing you can do — the clinical assessment of your own life.
You cannot heal what you refuse to diagnose.
Look at the number. Say it out loud if you need to. Then turn to the next page.

The Book That Changed My Financial Life

I want to tell you about the resource that, for me, became what a great attending physician is for a new resident: the voice that cut through the noise, named the problem plainly, and gave me a framework I could actually follow.

Dave Ramsey's Financial Peace University did not make me wealthy overnight. It did not eliminate my debt with a formula or a motivational speech. What it did was something more valuable: it gave me a language for money that I had never had. A sequence. A structure. A way of thinking about income and debt and savings and investment that was simple enough to actually implement — and rigorous enough to produce real results if you followed it with genuine commitment.

I was skeptical at first. I had encountered enough financial advice that felt designed for someone else's life — someone without student loans, without family obligations spanning two continents, without the irregular income that comes from working multiple clinical roles. But Ramsey's core principles were not built on assumptions about privilege. They were built on the premise that almost anyone, starting from almost anywhere, can change the trajectory of their financial life — if they are willing to accept the truth of where they are and commit to a different way of operating.

That premise I believed. Because I had already proven it was possible in my own career. I came to America with an IT background, pivoted to nursing, earned my BSN and then my MSN, and built an executive career, step by intentional step. Financial transformation was the same kind of work. Not glamorous. Not fast. But entirely possible.

THE 7 BABY STEPS — Dave Ramsey's Financial Peace University

The framework that started my financial transformation:

Step 1: Save $1,000 as a starter emergency fund — immediately

Step 2: Pay off all debt (except the mortgage) using the Debt Snowball

Step 3: Save 3–6 months of expenses as a fully funded emergency fund

Step 4: Invest 15% of household income into retirement accounts

Step 5: Save for your children's college fund

Step 6: Pay off your home early

Step 7: Build wealth and give generously

Note from Caroline: The Baby Steps are a starting framework, not a rigid religion. Adapt them to your clinical income, your family obligations, and your specific debt load. But the core principle — get out of consumer debt before you try to build wealth — is sound. Do not skip this step.

I am not telling you that Financial Peace University is the only path, or that Dave Ramsey's specific advice applies perfectly to every nurse reading this book. What I am telling you is this: find your version of this resource. Find the financial framework that gives you language, sequence, and accountability. Whether it is Financial Peace University, a financial coach, a trusted mentor, or a combination of tools, the point is that financial literacy is not self-generating. You have to seek it, actively and intentionally, and then apply what you learn with the same discipline you brought to passing your boards.

The Student Loan Question Every Nurse Should Ask

Let me address something that is rarely discussed with sufficient directness in conversations about nursing finances: the decision about student loans.

Here is my position, earned through experience rather than theory: if you can pay your tuition out of pocket — through income, through employer tuition assistance, through family support, through any means that does not require you to borrow — do that. Leave the student loan alone. Do not take it simply because it is available, simply because everyone else is taking it, or simply because it feels like the path of least resistance.

Student loans are not free money. They are deferred debt with interest that begins compounding the moment the money is disbursed, and they follow you with a tenacity that most other forms of debt do not. I have watched nurses carry student loan balances well into their forties and fifties — not because they were irresponsible borrowers, but because no one sat them down before graduation and explained the full cost of what they were signing.

The math is not complicated once you see it clearly. A loan of forty-seven thousand dollars at a six percent interest rate, on a standard ten-year repayment plan, costs nearly sixteen thousand dollars in interest alone. That is sixteen thousand dollars that will not go toward an emergency fund, a rental property, a retirement account, or your child's education. That is sixteen thousand dollars that goes to a lender in exchange for the privilege of borrowing money; you could perhaps have found another way to access it.

The Student Loan Decision Framework

BEFORE taking any student loan, ask these questions honestly:

1. Can I pay this tuition cost — even partially — without borrowing?
2. Has my employer offered tuition reimbursement or advancement?
3. Am I eligible for grants, scholarships, or institutional aid I have not applied for?
4. If I do borrow, do I understand the total repayment cost — not just the monthly payment?
5. Am I borrowing the maximum available, or only what I genuinely need?

The best student loan is the one you never took. The second best is the smallest one possible.-

For nurses already carrying student loan debt, your strategy depends on your loan type, income, and employer. Federal loans may qualify for income-driven repayment plans that cap your monthly payment based on what you earn. If you work for a nonprofit hospital or qualifying healthcare organization, Public Service Loan Forgiveness may eliminate your remaining balance after ten years of qualifying payments — a benefit that is worth investigating immediately if you have not already. Do not pay more than you legally owe, and do not ignore the programs designed to help you.

Credit Cards: The Tool That Became a Trap

I have a complicated relationship with credit cards. I think most nurses do.

We came to them in a moment of need — furnishing an apartment, covering a gap between paychecks, managing an unexpected expense. We used them because they were available and because no one had taught us to fear interest rates with the specificity they deserve. And then we watched the balance grow with a quiet horror that is very difficult to describe to someone who has not experienced it: the sense of a financial tide moving against you, slowly but persistently, in a direction you did not choose.

Here is what I know now that I did not know then: a credit card is a tool. Like any clinical instrument, its safety and its utility depend entirely on how it is used. Used correctly — paid in full each month, maintained at a low utilization rate, selected carefully for terms and benefits — a credit card can support your financial life without costing you anything. Used improperly, it is one of the most expensive forms of consumer debt.

Credit Utilization: The Number Most People Ignore

Your credit utilization ratio is the percentage of your available credit that you are currently using. If you have a card with a $3,000 limit and carry a $1,500 balance, your utilization is fifty percent. Credit scoring models generally reward utilization below 30%, and people with the strongest credit scores typically keep it below 10%.

This matters beyond your credit score. High utilization is a signal — to lenders, to yourself — that you are living beyond what you can comfortably sustain. Monitoring your utilization is not a vanity metric. It is a real-time indicator of your financial health, as useful in its way as a patient's vital signs.

Utilization Range	Impact on Credit	What It Signals
Under 10%	Excellent — actively helps score	Financially comfortable, intentional spender
10% – 30%	Good — minimal negative impact	Manageable debt, within sustainable limits
30% – 50%	Fair — begins to drag score	Possible strain; monitor closely
50% – 75%	Poor — significant score damage	Living beyond means; needs immediate attention
Above 75%	Damaging — major red flag	Financial crisis signal; urgent intervention needed

High Interest Rates and Annual Fees: The Two Red Lines

There are two features on a credit card that should function as automatic disqualifiers when you are in debt-elimination mode: a high interest rate and an annual fee.

A high interest rate — anything above fifteen percent, and many cards carry rates of twenty to twenty-nine percent — means that every month you carry a balance, a significant portion of your minimum payment goes to the lender rather than reducing what you owe. You can make payments faithfully for months and see your balance barely move because the interest is consuming most of what you are paying. This is not a malfunction. This is the product working exactly as designed — for the bank.

Annual fees are a separate problem. There are credit cards that charge annual fees of ninety-five dollars, two hundred and fifty dollars, or more — in exchange for rewards programs and travel benefits that make financial sense only if you have the disposable income to use them without carrying a balance. If you are in debt, you are paying an annual fee for the privilege of paying interest. That is a cost with no offsetting benefit.

Cards to Avoid When You Are Building Out of Debt

Any card with an APR above 20% — the interest will outpace your payments

Any card with an annual fee, unless the benefits clearly exceed the cost

Store-specific cards (retail, airline-branded) — typically high rates, limited utility

Cards that offer 'deferred interest' promotions — these can retroactively charge interest on the full original balance

Any card marketed with urgency or approval guarantees is a sign of predatory terms

The best credit card for someone eliminating debt is one with a low APR, no annual fee, and no temptation.

The Myth of More Credit Lines

Here is something I needed to be told plainly, and I am going to tell it to you the same way: having many open lines of credit is not financial sophistication. It is not a sign of prosperity. It is not a strategy — unless you are operating a business that requires access to capital, understand how to leverage business debt as a growth instrument, and have the financial discipline and systems to manage it without letting it consume you.

For the individual nurse trying to build financial stability, multiple open credit lines create multiple opportunities for balances to accumulate, multiple minimum payments to manage, and a complex web of utilization ratios that is easy to lose track of. The psychological effect alone is significant: when you have six or seven open accounts with varying balances and rates, the cognitive load of managing them becomes a form of financial chaos that makes intentional decision-making much harder.

I have watched nurses open new cards to transfer balances — a legitimate strategy when executed correctly — and then proceed to charge the original card back up, effectively doubling their debt while believing they were managing it. I have seen nurses apply for multiple cards in a short period, damaging their credit scores through hard inquiries, and then not understand why their scores dropped when they had been trying to improve them.

More credit lines do not make you more powerful. More credit lines make more opportunities for debt to grow silently in the dark.

The Exception: Business Debt

There is a meaningful distinction between consumer debt and business debt — and understanding that distinction is part of becoming a financially sophisticated healthcare professional.

Business debt, used strategically, is a lever. When I co-founded Icon Oncology Supply, access to credit and capital was not a lifestyle expense — it was a growth instrument. Money borrowed to purchase inventory that generates revenue, to establish infrastructure that supports a business model, to fund the operating costs of a company that produces income — this is a fundamentally different animal from a credit card balance that exists because the month's expenses exceeded the month's income.

The distinction is purpose and return. Consumer debt costs you money. Well-structured business debt, in a viable business, generates a return that exceeds its cost. Learning to think about debt in these terms — as either a liability or a calculated instrument — is one of the most important intellectual shifts in this entire book.

But that shift comes after you have dealt with the consumer debt. You cannot intelligently manage business capital if you are still paying 23% interest on furniture you purchased 3 years ago. Get out of consumer debt first. Then we will talk about leverage.

The Snowball, the Avalanche, and the One That Works for You

There are two primary strategies for eliminating multiple debts, and the debate between their proponents has been ongoing in personal finance circles for decades. I am going to describe both—and then tell you what I actually believe.

The Debt Snowball

The Debt Snowball, popularized by Dave Ramsey, works like this: list all your debts from smallest balance to largest, regardless of interest rate. Make minimum payments on everything. Put every extra dollar toward the smallest balance until it is gone. Then take what you were paying on that debt and roll it into the next smallest. And so on, until the list is empty.

The logic is psychological as much as mathematical. Eliminating small debts quickly generates momentum — the genuine, felt experience of winning — that sustains the discipline required to keep going through the larger, slower battles. For many people, this is not a small thing. The motivation to continue is itself a financial resource.

The Debt Avalanche

The Debt Avalanche works differently: list all your debts from highest interest rate to lowest, regardless of balance. Minimum payments on everything, extra dollars toward the highest-rate debt first. Mathematically, this approach results in lower total interest paid. The numbers are unambiguous on this point.

The challenge is behavioral: you may spend months or years making aggressive payments on a large, high-interest debt before it is eliminated — and you may never experience the motivational payoff of a balance reaching zero. For people who need visible progress to sustain discipline, the Avalanche is theoretically superior but practically harder to stick with.

My Honest Advice: The One That Works Is the One You Do

Snowball: Best if you need motivational wins to stay consistent — eliminates small debts quickly

Avalanche: Best if you are analytically motivated and can sustain discipline without visible milestones

Hybrid: Start with a small Snowball win to build momentum, then switch to Avalanche for larger balances

The wrong strategy, applied consistently, beats the right strategy abandoned after three months.

Pick the approach that fits how your brain works. Then do not stop.

Live Within Your Means — And Know What That Actually Means

There is a phrase in personal finance that is so frequently used it has lost almost all meaning: live within your means. I want to restore its meaning, because it is the foundation of every other strategy in this book.

Living within your means is not about deprivation. It is not about coupon clipping, denying yourself every pleasure, or apologizing for wanting a good life. It is about this: the money going out must not exceed the money coming in. Not most months. Every month. Consistently. Without exception.

That sounds simple. For most of us, it is not. Because our means are complicated — irregular shift income, variable overtime, family obligations that do not follow a schedule, unexpected expenses that do not care about our budgets. Living within your means as a nurse requires a more sophisticated version of this principle than the one found in standard personal finance books, and I want to give it to you plainly.

Living Within Your Means — The Clinical Version

Know your baseline income: what you earn without overtime, without the second job, without the PRN shifts

Build your essential budget around that number — not your best month, your baseline month

Treat overtime and extra shifts as savings accelerators, not as core income

When extra income arrives, direct it before it disappears: 50% to debt, 30% to savings, 20% to living

Do not expand your lifestyle every time your income expands — this is called lifestyle inflation, and it is the silent killer of wealth

Every purchase above a set threshold (your choice — fifty dollars, one hundred dollars) gets a twenty-four-hour delay before execution

The goal is not to spend less. The goal is to spend intentionally.

Living within your means is also, I want to say this directly, a gift to yourself and to everyone who depends on you. When you are not carrying the weight of financial anxiety — the constant low-grade pressure of owing more than you have — you show up differently. As a clinician. As a parent. As a partner. As a person. Financial peace is not a luxury. It is a health outcome. And you deserve it.

Financial Support Is Ongoing — Not a Destination

One of the most important things I learned through Financial Peace University and through my own recovery from the debt cycle was this: financial literacy is not a course you complete and set aside. It is a practice. An ongoing, active, evolving commitment to understanding how money works and applying that understanding to the specific conditions of your life as they change.

The debt you eliminate in your thirties will not be the last financial challenge you face. Income will change. Family obligations will evolve. Unexpected expenses will arrive without warning. Business opportunities will present themselves. The financial landscape of your life will shift — and what will determine your outcomes is not the absence of those shifts, but the literacy to navigate them.

Seek ongoing financial education. Read. Listen. Find a financial advisor or planner who understands the specific dynamics of healthcare professionals — the irregular income, the benefit structures, the student loan landscape, the unique risks and opportunities of clinical entrepreneurship. Join communities of nurses who are building wealth. Talk about money with the people in your life — openly, honestly, without the shame that silence perpetuates.

The conversation about money that your family never had is the one you get to start. In your home. With your children. In your nursing unit. With your colleagues. You do not have to have it all figured out to have the conversation. You just have to be willing to start it.

> ***Financial peace is not a destination you arrive at. It is a practice you commit to — one intentional decision at a time, for the rest of your life.***

BOARDROOM MOMENT

Heal Your Wealth – Chapter 3 Reflection

Confronting debt requires honesty, a plan, and the willingness to change behavior—not just the numbers. Answer these questions with the same precision you bring to patient care.

1. List every debt you currently carry: the creditor, the balance, the interest rate, and the minimum monthly payment. Put them in order — smallest balance to largest. This is your Snowball list. You now have a sequence.
2. Pull out every credit card you currently hold. For each one, write down the APR and the annual fee. Any card with an APR above 20% or an annual fee you cannot justify should be on a plan for elimination once the balance is cleared.
3. What is your current credit utilization across all cards combined? If you do not know, calculate it now: total balances divided by total credit limits. If it is above 30%, that number is your first target.
4. Have you investigated Public Service Loan Forgiveness if you work at a nonprofit hospital? Have you reviewed your employer's tuition assistance benefit? This week, look up both. Write down what you find.
5. What is one spending pattern — one recurring expense, one habit, one automatic cost — that you could eliminate or reduce starting this month and redirect toward debt elimination? Name it specifically. Then do it.

Debt is a chapter, not a life sentence. You have made it through harder clinical rotations than this. You will make it through this, too.

— — —

In Chapter 4, we address the budget that falls apart every time your schedule changes — and build one that actually works for a clinician's life. Rotating shifts, overnight differentials, the PRN income that arrives without warning: all of it accounted for, in a system you can sustain.

Because the goal is not a perfect budget. The goal is a budget that still works in month seven, when motivation has faded, and discipline is the only thing left. That budget exists. We are going to build it together.

Continue to Chapter 4: Budgeting on Rotating Shifts

CHAPTER FOUR

Budgeting on Rotating Shifts

On the question that changes everything: can you live without the extra income — and do you want to?

I want to ask you a question that most financial books never ask, and I want you to sit with it before you answer.

If your situation demanded it — if an injury, an illness, a family emergency, or a deliberate choice required you to work the bare minimum — could you live on that income alone? Not comfortably. Not luxuriously. But sustainably. Without the second job. Without the overtime. Without the extra shifts that have quietly become as much a part of your life as the shifts themselves.

For most nurses in the debt cycle, the honest answer is no. The extra income is not supplemental. It has become structural. The lifestyle has expanded to absorb it, the obligations have been built around it, and removing it would not reveal a smaller, simpler financial life — it would reveal a crisis.

That discovery — the moment I asked myself this question and did not like my answer — was one of the most clarifying financial moments of my life. And the journey from that answer to another is what this chapter is about.

> ***Extra income is consoling. But comfort built on income you cannot sustain is not security — it is a debt to your future self.***

The Credential That Gave Me My Life Back

Becoming a nurse practitioner changed my clinical scope of practice. What I did not fully anticipate was how much it would change my relationship with time.

As an RN working rotating twelve-hour shifts, my schedule was largely fixed by the unit's needs. The hours were long, the rotation was demanding, and flexibility — true flexibility — was limited. The work was meaningful. The income was necessary. But the structure of the job made certain things nearly impossible: being reliably present for school pickups, attending events without the anxiety of a shift looming, building a daily rhythm that included my children as something other than a footnote squeezed between obligations.

The NP credential opened a different kind of clinical role — one with greater schedule flexibility, higher hourly earning potential, and, critically, greater control over the architecture of my professional life. It did not eliminate the work. It changed what the work required of me beyond the clinical hours. And that difference, which sounds abstract when you are still in the RN role looking toward it, becomes completely concrete the first morning you drop your child at school and arrive at work without the guilt of knowing you will not be there when they come home.

I want to be careful here because I am not saying that the NP credential is the path for every nurse. There are RNs who have built deeply intentional, financially sound, family-centered lives without advancing their degree. The credential is not the point. The intentionality is the point. What becoming an NP gave me was the specific vehicle for that intentionality. You will need to find yours.

To My Children

Every intentional decision I made was made with you in mind.

The downgraded apartment, the budget that required discipline, the school I went back to — all of it.

You were never the sacrifice. You were always the reason.

I hope that when you are old enough to read this, you know: being present for you was never negotiable.

The Peace That Money Cannot Buy — And the Budget That Protects It

There is a specific kind of peace that comes from picking your child up from school yourself.

I know how small that sounds on paper. In the context of a chapter on financial strategy, it might seem like a digression—a sentimental moment inserted between the practical frameworks. It is not. It is the entire point.

When I became intentional about my finances — when I built a budget that was honest about what I needed and stripped away what I had been financing out of habit or anxiety — the most profound result was not a number. It was time. The ability to be where my children were when it mattered. Not to be halfway through a twelve-hour shift, wondering who was picking them up, whether they were okay, and what I was missing. To drop them off in the morning and pick them up in the afternoon and be present for the hours in between — not because I had arranged a heroic logistical solution, but because I had built a financial life that did not require me to sell those hours to pay for it.

That peace — the knowing — outweighs any number I could have produced by working more. I say this as someone who has been on both sides of that equation, and I say it without any qualification: the time you spend with your children when they are small is time you cannot buy back. It does not compound. It does not accrue interest. It simply passes, and either you were there or you were not.

> ***Kids grow, and soon they are gone. The shift you picked up instead of being there will not remember you. They will.***

Building a budget that protects your time is not a soft goal. It is one of the most rigorous financial objectives a parent can pursue — because it requires you to be absolutely precise about what your life actually costs without the overtime, and then to build your income and expenses around that number with genuine discipline.

The budget I will help you build in this chapter is not a theoretical exercise. It is the specific financial architecture that makes presence possible. The one that lets you answer yes to the question I asked at the beginning of this chapter — yes, I could live on my baseline income if I had to — and mean it.

The Daycare Trap — The Math Nobody Runs

I have watched this scenario play out more times than I can count, among nurses I have worked alongside, mentored, and befriended across years of clinical practice. A nurse returns from maternity leave, full of determination to maintain her income and her career. She finds a daycare—a good one, because she will not compromise on her child's care—and runs the math to see if she can afford it. She looks at her take-home pay and the monthly daycare fee, and the numbers clear the line.

What she does not always run is the full arithmetic.

The True Cost of Full-Time Daycare: What the Monthly Fee Doesn't Include

Monthly daycare tuition (infant/toddler rates in many cities): $1,500 – $2,800+

Transportation to and from daycare: fuel, mileage, or rideshare costs

Work wardrobe maintenance: scrubs, shoes, and professional clothing that daycare days require

Convenience food spending: the meals not cooked on the days of exhaustion arrive with you

Sick day care: backup care when daycare is closed, or the child is ill

Late pickup fees: the ones that come on overtime days and long shift days

The emotional cost of the arrangement — harder to quantify, but real

In many cases, the net income from the shift — after all associated costs — is significantly smaller than the paycheck suggests.

In some cases, it is nearly zero. In a few cases, it is negative.

Run the full math before you decide that working more is the answer.

I am not arguing that nurses should not work or that career and parenthood are incompatible. They are absolutely compatible, and I am the proof of that. What I am arguing is that the financial decision to work a particular schedule — particularly the decision to add extra shifts or a second job — must be made on accurate numbers, not on the gross income the extra work produces without accounting for the costs it entails.

I have known nurses who worked 60-hour weeks for years, believing they were building financial security, who discovered, when they finally ran the numbers, that a meaningful portion of those additional hours was absorbed by the costs those hours generated. The childcare, the convenience spending, the physical and emotional recovery — all of it has a price. And that price does not appear on the pay stub.

Intentionality means running the full calculation. Not the comfortable one. The complete one.

Meaningful Work Should Not Cost You Your Family

This is the principle I want to state plainly, without qualification, because I believe it is true and I have seen too many nurses live as though it is not:

Career fulfillment and family presence are not competing values. They are not a trade-off you are required to make. The belief that meaningful work demands family sacrifice — that to be taken seriously as a clinician, a leader, or a professional, you must accept that your family gets what is left after the work is done — is a belief that the healthcare system has a long history of exploiting, particularly in its treatment of nurses, and particularly in its treatment of women.

You are allowed to build a clinical career that is rigorous, fulfilling, and significant — and to be home for dinner. You are allowed to pursue advanced credentials and executive leadership — and to attend the school play. You are allowed to be excellent at your work and excellent at your presence. These are not contradictions. They are the result of an intentional financial and professional architecture you build, rather than accepting the default one the system offers.

> ***Meaningful work and meaningful presence are not enemies. They are partners — if you build your financial life in a way that honors both.***

What makes this possible is the budget. Not the restrictive, punishing version of a budget that most people abandon after six weeks. The intentional version — the one that tells you exactly what your life costs at its sustainable baseline, protects the things that matter most to you from financial pressure, and gives you clear sight lines on where the extra income, when it comes, should actually go.

That is the budget we are going to build now.

Building a Budget That Works on Any Shift Schedule

Step One: Establish Your Baseline Income

Your baseline income is what you earn reliably — your guaranteed hours, your base rate, your contracted shifts — without overtime, without the second job, without PRN, without anything extra. This is the number your budget must be built around.

This is not the number most nurses use when they build a budget, which is precisely why most nurses' budgets fail. If you build your essential expenses around your best month's income and your best month includes three overtime shifts, you have created a budget that requires overtime to function. You have made overtime non-optional. You have handed the hospital the leverage to schedule you however they need, because you need every hour they offer.

Build around your guaranteed baseline. Everything above that is allocation, not lifestyle.

Step Two: Categorize Your Expenses With Brutal Honesty

Every expense in your life belongs to one of three categories: essential, intentional, and habitual. Essential expenses are non-negotiable — housing, food, utilities, insurance, minimum debt payments, and childcare if you are working. Intentional expenses are chosen consciously — the subscription you actually use, the membership that genuinely serves you, the experiences that matter to your family. Habitual expenses are the ones that happen automatically without conscious decision — the subscription you forgot was running, the convenience spending that adds up invisibly, the restaurant meals that belong to a lifestyle you built in a different financial season.

Most financial waste lives in the habitual category. Not in the big decisions — in the small, automatic ones that were never revisited after circumstances changed.

EXPENSE CATEGORY	Your Monthly Amount
— ESSENTIAL —	
Housing (rent or mortgage)	$
Utilities (electric, gas, water)	$
Phone	$
Groceries (realistic amount)	$
Transportation (car payment, insurance, gas)	$
Health insurance / medical costs	$
Childcare (if applicable)	$
Minimum debt payments (all)	$
Family obligations (remittances, support)	$

ESSENTIAL TOTAL	$
— INTENTIONAL —	
Subscriptions you actively use	$
Gym/wellness	$
Children's activities	$
Giving/tithing	$
INTENTIONAL TOTAL	$
— HABITUAL (review each one) —	
Subscriptions you forgot about	$
Dining out / convenience food	$
Impulse or unplanned purchases	$
HABITUAL TOTAL	$
GRAND TOTAL	$

Step Three: The Baseline Test

Subtract your Grand Total from your baseline income. If the number is positive, you have a workable budget. If it is negative, you have a gap — and that gap is the exact amount by which you are currently dependent on extra income to sustain your lifestyle. That number is not a judgment. It is your assignment.

The Baseline Test

Baseline Monthly Income (guaranteed hours only): $__________

Minus Total Monthly Expenses (from worksheet above): $__________

Result: $__________

If POSITIVE: You can live within your baseline. Extra income is a wealth-building tool.

If NEGATIVE: The gap is your number. This is what you are working to close—through expense reduction, not by working more hours.

Step Four: Allocate Extra Income Before It Arrives

When the overtime shift is approved, when the PRN payment lands, when the differential pays out — that money needs a destination before it hits your account. Because money without a destination finds its own way, and it rarely chooses debt payoff or investment without your instruction.

Here is a simple allocation framework for extra income, adapted for nurses in different financial stages:

Extra Income Allocation Framework

IF YOU ARE IN DEBT ELIMINATION MODE:

70% → Targeted debt payment (your Snowball or Avalanche list)
20% → Emergency fund (until 3 months of expenses saved)
10% → You (one intentional, guilt-free purchase — sustainability matters)

IF YOUR DEBT IS CLEARED AND BUILDING SAVINGS:

50% → Investment/retirement accounts
30% → Savings goals (property, education, emergency fund completion)
20% → You and your family (experiences, not things)

IF YOU ARE IN WEALTH-BUILDING MODE:

40% → Investment and income-producing assets
30% → Business or entrepreneurial reinvestment
20% → Savings and liquidity
10% → Giving — generosity is a wealth habit, not a luxury

The exact percentages are less important than the practice of deciding in advance.

The Shift Schedule Is Not Fixed — Your Life Can Be

One of the most disempowering beliefs in nursing is the idea that the schedule is simply what it is — that the rotating shifts, the mandatory overtime, the weekend rotations, the on-call requirements are conditions of employment rather than points to negotiate. For many nurses, particularly early in their careers, this feels true. The unit needs what it needs, and the nurse provides it.

But as you build clinical experience, advance your credentials, demonstrate value, and develop a financial baseline that does not require every available shift, something changes: you begin to have leverage. Not unlimited leverage. Not leverage that erases the demands of the profession. But the quiet leverage of a clinician who does not desperately need the extra hours — and who therefore has more ability to shape which hours they work.

Financial intentionality is professional leverage. When you are not living paycheck to paycheck, you can decline the shift that conflicts with your child's recital without the weight of financial panic. You can take the position that offers more flexibility and slightly less income without catastrophic consequences to your budget. You can make career decisions based on fit, values, and growth rather than exclusively on the size of the paycheck — because your baseline budget has made a range of incomes viable rather than requiring the maximum at all times.

> ***When you do not desperately need every extra shift, you stop being owned by the schedule. That freedom is worth more than the shift's pay.***

To the Nurse Watching Her Paycheck Disappear Into Daycare

I want to speak directly to the nurse who is doing the math right now — who is working forty-eight or sixty hours a week, watching the daycare invoice arrive, and feeling the quiet, exhausting arithmetic of it all. The one who loves her work and loves her children and is trying to hold both without losing either.

You are not doing it wrong. You are doing it in a system that was not designed with you in mind — a system that requires dual incomes to afford housing in the cities where hospitals are located, that provides minimal parental leave, that schedules shifts in patterns that make consistent childcare planning nearly impossible, and that has never fully reckoned with the fact that the majority of its nursing workforce is made up of mothers.

I am not asking you to solve the system. I am asking you to build a financial life within it that protects what you cannot replace: the time with your children while they are small. That means running the full math on the extra shifts. It means asking honestly whether the income they produce is worth what they cost — in dollars, in energy, in hours. It means designing your budget around presence rather than income, and then finding an income structure that serves that budget.

It is not easy. Nothing in this book is easy. But it is possible. And the nurses who figure it out do not regret it. Not one.

What Presence Costs — And What It Returns

The school pickup costs you: one shift you did not take, income you did not earn.

The school pickup returns: a moment your child will carry forward. Presence they will feel even when they are too young to name it.

The budget that makes it possible costs you: discipline, intentionality, and the willingness to live below your maximum income.

The budget returns: peace. Options. The specific freedom of not needing every dollar that exists.

Intentionality Is the Budget's Operating System

Every practical tool in this chapter — the baseline test, the expense categories, the extra income allocation framework, the shift leverage principle — is only as effective as the intention behind it. A budget is not a spreadsheet. A budget is a set of values expressed in numbers. It tells you, more honestly than almost any other document in your life, what you have actually decided matters.

When I became intentional about time with my children — when I stopped treating their hours as the residual of my schedule and started treating my schedule as something I built around their hours — my budget had to change to reflect that. Not because I became less ambitious professionally. Because I became clear about what the ambition was actually for.

The money is for the life. Not the other way around.

That is the sentence I want you to carry with you in every financial decision you make from this chapter forward. The budget exists to protect the life you are building. The shifts exist to fund the budget. The career exists to give you the platform, the income, and the fulfillment that make a fully lived life possible. In that order.

When the order gets reversed — when the life exists to support the career that supports the budget — the budget is no longer a tool. It has become a cage. And the nurses who walk away from this book with something different are the ones who learn to tell the difference.

The money is for the life. Not the other way around. Hold that sentence. It will make every budget decision easier.

BOARDROOM MOMENT

Heal Your Wealth — Chapter 4 Reflection

A budget is not a punishment. It is a permission structure—the document that tells your money where to go so it stops disappearing without your consent. Answer these questions, then build your baseline budget below.

6. Complete the expense worksheet in this chapter using your actual monthly figures. Then run the Baseline Test: subtract your essential and intentional expenses from your guaranteed baseline income. What is the number? If it is negative, that gap is your most urgent financial assignment. If it is positive, you have building material.
7. How much of your current lifestyle is funded by income you cannot guarantee — overtime, PRN shifts, a second job? If that income disappeared tomorrow, what specifically would you cut? The answer tells you what is essential and what is optional.
8. If you have children: run the full daycare arithmetic. Include transportation, convenience food, backup care costs, and the energy cost you would assign a dollar value to if you could. Does the math still show that the extra shifts are the right answer? What does the honest calculation tell you?
9. What does presence mean to you specifically — not abstractly, but in concrete terms? Name one recurring moment with your children or family that you have missed because of work that you would not miss again if your financial life were structured differently.
10. Write your intentionality statement: 'I am building my financial life so that I can ___________.' Complete that sentence with something specific, personal, and true. This is your budget's operating system. Put it somewhere you will see it when the discipline gets hard.

Your time is your most finite resource. Your budget is how you protect it.

— — —

In Chapter 5, we address the trap in full: the second job, the overtime cycle, and the specific strategies for breaking free from trading time for income that does not compound. You have already identified the gap that the extra income is filling. Now we talk about what fills that gap instead — intentionally, sustainably, and without working seven days a week to do it.

Because you did not become a nurse practitioner, or an executive, or an entrepreneur, or pick up this book, to spend the rest of your career running on someone else's schedule. You did it to build something. Let's talk about what that something looks like — and how to get there without giving up the life you are building it for.

Continue to Chapter 5: The Second Job & The Overtime Trap

CHAPTER FIVE

The Second Job & The Overtime Trap

Take overtime when you want to — not when you must to survive

Seven days a week.

I have known nurses who worked seven days a week for months at a stretch. Not because they loved the hospital that much. Not because the work was so compelling that they could not stay away. But because the math of their lives had closed around them so tightly that stopping — even for one day — felt like a financial risk they could not absorb. The debt was real. The bills were real. The gap between what came in and what went out was real. And overtime was the only instrument they had found to bridge it.

I understand this intimately, because I lived a version of it. Two hospitals. Back-to-back shifts. The specific exhaustion of a body that has been on its feet for twelve hours, arriving somewhere else to be on its feet for twelve more. The way fatigue becomes a kind of background noise after a while — not loud enough to stop you, just loud enough to make everything harder. The way you stop asking whether this is sustainable and start asking only whether this paycheck will cover what was left unresolved last week.

But here is what I also know, from the other side of that season: all of it — every extra shift, every second job, every Saturday surrendered to a time clock — produced almost nothing permanent. Because I was not intentional with what I was earning. I was earning to spend, spending to cope, and coping to get through the week so I could earn again. The revolving door was not the overtime itself. The revolving door was the relationship between the earning and the spending that no amount of hours could outrun.

> ***You can work seven days a week and still end the month exactly where you started. The problem was never the hours. It was what happened to them.***

The Revolving Door of Debt

Let me describe the mechanics of the overtime trap clearly, because understanding exactly how it works is the first step to walking out of it.

You are short on money. You pick up an extra shift. The extra shift pays out, and you cover the immediate gap—the credit card minimum, the overdue bill, the expense that arrived without warning. Relief. Brief, genuine relief.

And then something happens that you did not plan for, because you were too exhausted to plan: the income expands your sense of what is available. Not dramatically. Subtly. The grocery cart is slightly fuller. The takeout order happens one more night that week because you worked six days and don't have the bandwidth to cook. You pick up something small that you genuinely needed and had been putting off. None of these decisions feels significant in isolation. Together, they absorb the extra shift.

The following month, the same gap appears. Because the lifestyle that generated the gap last month is still intact — in some cases, slightly larger. So, you pick up another extra shift. And the cycle continues, with an efficiency so quiet and so consistent that it can go on for years without ever announcing itself as the crisis it is.

This is the revolving door. It does not announce itself. It does not feel dramatic. It simply keeps turning, month after month, keeping you in motion while delivering you back to the same place you started.

Signs You Are in the Overtime Revolving Door

You cannot remember the last time you worked only your contracted hours

Your budget is built around income that requires overtime to be accurate

When you decline an extra shift, you feel financial anxiety — not relief

Your bank balance looks the same at the end of overtime months as regular months

You are tired in a way that sleep does not fully address

The idea of working less feels impossible, not optional

You have not had a full, unscheduled weekend in longer than you can remember

If three or more of these are true: you are not using overtime. Overtime is using you.

What the Extra Shift Actually Costs

We talked in Chapter 4 about running the full arithmetic on extra work. Here, I want to go deeper—not just the financial cost of the additional hours, but the full cost. Because the overtime trap is not only a money problem, it is a life problem that shows up as a money problem.

The Financial Cost

Every hour of overtime you work above a certain threshold is taxed at your marginal rate — which means the further into overtime you go, the smaller the net gain per hour. A nurse earning a significant base salary who picks up consistent overtime may find that twenty to thirty percent or more of each overtime dollar goes to taxes before it ever reaches her account. The gross number on the pay stub is not the number that matters.

The net number — after taxes, after the costs the shift generates — is the number that matters.

THE REAL OVERTIME CALCULATION	
Overtime gross pay (per shift)	$
Minus taxes (estimated 25–35% marginal rate)	- $
Minus childcare or backup care cost	- $
Minus convenience food/meals (too tired to cook)	- $
Minus transportation extra costs	- $
Minus any work-related expenses	- $
NET INCOME FROM EXTRA SHIFT	= $
Is this number worth what the shift costs you in hours, energy, and presence?	Answer honestly.

The Physical Cost

Nursing is one of the most physically demanding professions in existence. Twelve-hour shifts require sustained physical activity — prolonged standing, patient transfers, repetitive motion — at an intensity that accumulates damage over time. The research on nurse fatigue is unambiguous: error rates increase, reaction times slow, and the risk of on-the-job injury rises with consecutive long shifts. You are not just tired at the end of a seven-day stretch. You are a different clinician — slower, less precise, more prone to the kind of mistakes that a rested version of you would not make.

There is a cost to that. To your patients. To your license. To your career longevity. And to your body, which will eventually present a bill for what you borrowed from it during those years of maximum output — in the form of chronic pain, burnout, adrenal fatigue, and the specific kind of depletion that does not respond to a long weekend.

The Invisible Cost

The invisible cost is the hardest to quantify and the most important to name: the cost of who you are not being while you are at the second job. The parent who is not present. The partner who is too depleted to connect. The friend who keeps rescheduling. The person who wanted a full life, somewhere along the way, started living only the working part of it.

These are not small costs. They compound, like debt, in ways that are difficult to see in the moment and impossible to miss in retrospect. The nurse who worked through her children's early years because she had to will have a reckoning with that choice — not necessarily one of regret, but of reckoning. The nurse who works through them when she does not have to is making a choice whose cost will become clear in a currency that cannot be earned back.

> ***Your body keeps the score of every shift you worked past what it needed. Your family keeps the score of every hour you were gone when you didn't have to be. Both accounts come due.***

Intentional Spending: The Exit from the Revolving Door

The solution to the overtime trap is not to stop working hard. It is to become intentional with what the work produces.

Intentional spending is not restrictive spending. It is not the joyless version of financial discipline where you deny yourself everything in pursuit of a number. It is spending that you have chosen — consciously, specifically, in alignment with the financial life you are building — rather than spending that simply happens because the money was available and the habit was already formed.

The difference between a nurse who works overtime and builds wealth and a nurse who works overtime and stays in debt is rarely the amount they earn. It is what they do with the earnings between the shifts. One has a plan that the income serves. The other has income that is spent outpacing it, regardless of how many hours it takes to generate it.

The Intentional Spending Test — Ask Before Every Non-Essential Purchase

1. Is this purchase aligned with the financial life I am building?
2. Am I buying this because I want it, or because I am recovering from a hard week?
3. If I did not have overtime income this month, would I still buy this?
4. Does this purchase move me toward my freedom number, or further from it?
5. Will I remember this purchase in six months, or will it have disappeared into the background?

You do not need to answer yes to all five. But you should be able to answer at least three.

If you cannot, put it down and come back in twenty-four hours.

Intentionality is not the absence of spending. It is the presence of decision.

I am not asking you to stop spending on things that bring genuine value to your life. I am asking you to stop spending unconsciously — on the takeout that happens out of exhaustion rather than desire, on the purchase that fills a moment rather than serves a goal, on the subscription that renews because canceling it requires an energy you do not currently have. That spending — the automatic, the habitual, the comfort-seeking — is what feeds the revolving door. And it is entirely within your power to stop it.

The Difference Between Want and Must

Here is the sentence that changed how I thought about overtime permanently: take it when you want to, not when you must to survive.

Read that again, slowly. Because there is a world of difference between those two conditions — and living in one versus the other is not primarily a matter of income. It is a matter of financial architecture.

When overtime is something you do because you want to — because you have a specific financial goal, the extra income will accelerate, because you find genuine satisfaction in the clinical work, because the opportunity is meaningful and the timing is right — it is a tool. A powerful one. An extra shift in that context is a choice that adds to your life rather than taking from it.

When overtime is something you do because you must — because the bills are already stretched, because the credit card needs addressing before the next cycle, because your budget cannot close without those additional hours — it is a trap. You have ceded the decision to your circumstances. The hospital knows it. Your body knows it. And somewhere underneath the exhaustion, you know it too.

Two Nurses, Same Shift — Different Realities

NURSE A — Overtime by necessity:

Works an extra shift because this month's expenses exceeded income.

Takes home $X after taxes. Covers the gap. Feels relief — briefly.

Next month, the gap reappears. The cycle continues.

Overtime is mandatory. Declining feels impossible. The schedule owns her.

NURSE B — Overtime by choice:

Works an extra shift because she has a target: eliminating her last credit card.

Takes home the same $X. Sends 100% to the card. Watches the balance drop.

Next month, she declines the extra shift. Takes her daughter to the museum instead.

Overtime is optional. Saying yes means something because saying no is equally available.

Same credential. Same shift. Same pay. Completely different lives.

The difference is a budget that works without overtime.

Breaking Free — The Practical Path Out

The path from overtime by necessity to overtime by choice is not instant. It is a sequence. And like every clinical protocol, it works because of the order as much as the individual steps.

Phase One: Stop the Leak

Before the extra income can build anything, the spending leak must be addressed. Go back to your expense worksheet from Chapter 4 and find the habitual spending — the automatic, the unconscious, the comfort-seeking. Calculate what it costs you monthly. That number is the first number to reclaim. You do not earn your way out of a leak. You fix the leak.

Phase Two: Build the Floor

The floor is your baseline budget—the one we built in Chapter 4, covering only essential and intentional expenses on guaranteed income. Once you know your floor, you know exactly how much overtime is structurally required. If the answer is zero, you are already free. If the answer is positive, that specific number is your target — not the shift count, not the hours, but the exact dollar amount you need to close the gap through expense reduction, income optimization, or both.

Phase Three: Give Every Overtime Dollar a Destination

Once you are working from a baseline budget that functions without overtime, every extra dollar earned through additional shifts becomes a wealth-building instrument rather than a survival mechanism. It goes somewhere specific before it arrives. Debt elimination. Emergency fund. Investment account. Down payment. College fund. Not to the general account, where the lifestyle will absorb it without ceremony.

This is the single habit that separates nurses who build wealth from nurses who earn significant incomes and have little to show for it a decade later. The overtime is the same. The destination is different. And the destination is everything.

Phase Four: Protect Your Rest as a Financial Asset

This may be the most unconventional advice in this chapter, but I believe it deeply: your rest is a financial asset. A rested nurse makes better clinical decisions, sustains her career longer, avoids the burnout that forces career interruptions, and shows up as a better manager, leader, and entrepreneur when those opportunities present themselves. The nurse who is perpetually depleted has narrowed her options — not just personally, but professionally. You cannot build a business, pursue a promotion, or think strategically about your financial future when your baseline is exhaustion.

Protecting your days off is not laziness. It is the maintenance of the asset that generates everything else.

> ***Rest is not the reward for finishing all the work. There will always be more work. Rest is the strategy that makes the work sustainable — and the wealth possible.***

The Second Job: When It Makes Sense and When It Does Not

A second job can be a legitimate and powerful financial strategy. I want to be clear about that, because this chapter is not an argument against earning more. It is an argument for earning more intentionally.

The second job makes sense when it has a specific, time-limited purpose. You are eliminating a specific debt. You are building an emergency fund in a compressed timeline. You are funding a credential or a business investment that will change your earning trajectory. In these cases, the second job is a sprint — a defined period of higher output in service of a specific goal, with an end date built in.

The second job does not make sense when it is structural — when it exists to fund a lifestyle that has expanded to require it, when it has no end date, when the income it produces is absorbed before it can accomplish anything permanent. In that case, it is not a strategy. It is a subsidy for a spending pattern that needs to change.

SECOND JOB — STRATEGIC	SECOND JOB — STRUCTURAL
Has a specific goal attached	Exists to cover general expenses
Has a defined end date	Has been ongoing for over a year with no exit plan
Extra income goes to a named destination	Extra income disappears into the budget
You could stop it without a financial crisis	Stopping it would create an immediate crisis
You chose it — it serves you	You need it — it owns you
Energizing because purposeful	Draining because indefinite

Ask yourself, honestly, which column describes your current situation. If the answer is the right column, the work is not to work harder. The work is to redesign the budget—and possibly the lifestyle—so that the structural dependency becomes a strategic choice.

What Freedom Actually Looks Like

I want to tell you what it felt like the first time I declined an overtime shift and felt nothing but relief.

Not guilt. Not anxiety. Not the quiet calculation of what the missing hours would cost me. Just relief. The clean, spacious feeling of an unscheduled day that belonged entirely to me and to the people I had built my financial life to protect time for.

That feeling is available to you. It is not a personality trait or a financial privilege reserved for people who earn more than you do. It is the result of a budget that tells the truth, an expense structure aligned with your actual values, and an income that covers the life you have intentionally designed. It is buildable. It is yours to build.

You may be at the beginning of that building right now — in the middle of debt elimination, or just beginning to see the gap between your baseline and your overtime-dependent budget close. The feeling of freedom is not at the end of the process. It arrives in increments, each time you make an intentional choice, each time you decline something because you want to rather than because you cannot afford it, each time the overtime becomes a tool rather than a lifeline.

The Goal Is Not More Hours — The Goal Is This

To wake up on a Saturday and choose whether to work — not be forced to.

To pick up an extra shift because it accelerates a goal you have named and claimed.

To look at your bank balance at the end of a month without overtime and see that it held.

To be tired sometimes because the work is meaningful — not because survival demanded it.

That is the life this chapter is building toward. And it starts with the next decision you make.

A Word to the Nurse Who Cannot Stop Yet

I know that some of you reading this chapter are not yet in a position to decline the overtime. The obligations are real. The debt is real. The family back home is real. The gap between the baseline and the bills is real, and the extra shifts are the only bridge available right now.

I am not asking you to stop. I am asking you to start.

Start by running the real arithmetic on every extra shift you pick up. Start by giving the extra income a specific destination rather than letting it disappear into the general account. Start by identifying the one expense — just one — that feeds the cycle and eliminating it this month. Start by doing the baseline test from Chapter 4 and knowing precisely what gap you are bridging.

The shift from necessity to choice is not made in a single decision. It is made in a hundred small ones, over months, each one nudging the gap a little narrower. You are not trying to transform everything at once. You are trying to make the next decision better than the last one. That is enough. That is exactly enough.

> ***You do not have to solve the whole thing today. You just have to make the next decision intentionally. One decision, repeated with discipline, is how every financial transformation begins.***

BOARDROOM MOMENT

Heal Your Wealth — Chapter 5 Reflection

These questions are designed to move you from survival mode to strategic mode. Answer them honestly — with a pen, not in your head.

11. In the past three months, how many extra shifts or overtime hours have you worked? Now calculate: where did that income go? Be specific. If you cannot account for it, that is your answer — and your starting point.
12. Is your current overtime strategic or structural? Use the two-column table in this chapter to be honest. If it is structural, name the one expense change that would begin to shift it.
13. Complete the Real Overtime Calculation table for one recent extra shift. After taxes and associated costs, what did you actually net? Was that amount worth what the shift cost you in hours, energy, and presence?
14. Write down the specific goal your next overtime shift will serve. Not 'bills' — something specific. A named debt. A savings target. An investment account contribution. A defined amount. If you cannot name it, wait until you can.
15. What would you do with a free Saturday — a full, unscheduled, unhurried Saturday — if your finances did not require you to fill it with work? Write it down in detail. That vision is your reason. Hold onto it.

Overtime by choice is a wealth accelerator. Overtime by necessity is a trap. The goal of this chapter is to make it always the former, never the latter.

— — —

In Chapter 6, we move from surviving to growing. You have built a budget, confronted debt, and begun to reclaim your time from the overtime trap. Now it is time to talk about what happens to money when you stop spending it and start deploying it — the basics of investing that nobody taught in nursing school, demystified and made practical for the clinician's specific financial life.

Because healing your wealth was never only about getting out of debt, it was about building something. Something that grows while you sleep, while you are present for your children, while you are doing the work you trained for — without needing you to trade every available hour to sustain it.

That is what investing is. And it is closer than you think.

Continue to Chapter 6: Investing 101 in Scrubs

CHAPTER SIX

Investing 101 in Scrubs

Start small. Use every tool available. Build something that works while you rest.

There is a lesson I learned on the hospital floor that nobody taught in a classroom, and it applies as much to investing as it does to clinical practice: what you look like is far less important than what you actually do.

I have worked alongside nurses in the finest designer scrubs who delivered mediocre care, and nurses in plain, worn sets who were the most precise and compassionate clinicians on the unit. The scrubs were never the indicator. The cleanliness was. The professionalism was. The knowledge, the presence, the discipline — those were the indicators. The brand on the fabric was irrelevant.

Money works the same way. The appearance of wealth — the designer bag, the luxury car, the expensive apartment in the prestigious building — is not wealth. It is the costume of wealth, worn by people who are often spending at a level that prevents the real thing from ever arriving. True investing is quiet. It does not announce itself. It compounds in the background while you are focused on living, and it shows up eventually not as a possession but as an option — the freedom to choose, to slow down, to not need the next shift.

This chapter is about building that quiet, compounding reality. Starting from where you actually are, with what you actually have, using every resource available to you — beginning with the ones your employer is already offering and you may not yet be fully using.

> ***Wealth is not what you wear. Wealth is what you build — quietly, consistently, in the spaces between the things that are visible.***

Investing in Meaningful Work First

Before we talk about stocks and retirement accounts, I want to make an argument that most investing books skip entirely: the first and most important investment you will ever make is in your own clinical competence and professional positioning.

Comfortable, quality scrubs are not vanity — they are a tool. A physically comfortable nurse, professionally confident in her appearance, and appropriately equipped for her role, shows up differently than one who is distracted by discomfort or undermined by clothing that does not support the work. This is intentional investment at its most basic: spending money on what genuinely supports your capacity to perform, rather than on what impresses others or fills an emotional gap.

The same principle extends to every professional investment: the certification that expands your scope of practice, the conference that puts you in a room with people whose thinking will sharpen yours, the textbook that deepens your clinical knowledge, the coach or mentor whose perspective accelerates your growth. These are investments. They generate returns — in earning power, in opportunity, in the credibility that opens the next door.

Invest in your competence first. Invest in your comfort as a professional. Then invest the financial returns that competence generates into the instruments that will multiply them.

The Nurse Who Invests in Herself First

She buys quality scrubs that last three years, not cheap ones that last three months.

She pays for the certification, which increases her hourly rate by $8.

She attends the conference that connects her to the opportunity she could not have found alone.

Every dollar spent on her own capacity is a dollar invested at the highest possible return.

This is where intentional investment begins — not in a brokerage account, but in the person who will manage one.

Start Small — The Permission You Have Been Waiting For

One of the most damaging myths in personal finance is the idea that investing requires a substantial initial investment. It does not. It requires a decision and a start date.

I know nurses who waited years to begin investing because they were waiting to have enough to make it feel meaningful. Meanwhile, the nurses who started with fifty dollars a month — who set up an automatic contribution and forgot about it — had been compounding quietly for years before the waiters made their first move. The difference in their outcomes a decade later was not explained by income. It was explained by the start date.

Compound interest is the most powerful financial force available to someone with time and patience — and nurses, by the nature of their training, understand time and patience intimately. The principle is simple: the money you invest earns returns. Those returns are reinvested and earn returns of their own. Over time, the growth accelerates — not because you invested more, but because the existing investment has been working longer. Starting with a small amount early is almost always more powerful than starting with a large amount late.

The Power of Starting – A Simple Illustration

Nurse A starts investing $200/month at age 28. Stops at 38. Never invests another dollar.
Nurse B waits. Starts investing $200/month at age 38. Continues until age 65.

At age 65, assuming a 7% average annual return:
Nurse A (invested for 10 years, then stopped): approximately $400,000+
Nurse B (invested for 27 years, started late): approximately $340,000+

Nurse A invested LESS total money—and ended up with MORE.
The variable that determined the outcome was not the amount. It was the start date.

Start today. With whatever you have. The clock is already running.

Maximize What Your Employer Is Already Offering

Before you open a brokerage account, before you research individual stocks, before you make any independent investment decision — go back to your HR portal and read your benefits summary with the eyes of someone who now understands what is at stake.

Employer-sponsored retirement accounts — the 403(b) for nonprofit hospital employees, the 401(k) for for-profit systems — are among the most powerful wealth-building tools available to healthcare professionals. Not because the investment options inside them are extraordinary, but because of the match.

When your employer offers to match your contributions — even partially, even up to a small percentage of your salary — that match is a 100% immediate return on the dollars you contribute up to that threshold. No stock, no index fund, no investment product of any kind can reliably guarantee an immediate 100% return. And yet an enormous number of nurses are not contributing enough to capture their full match. Some are not contributing at all.

The Most Common and Costly Investing Mistake in Nursing

Not contributing enough to your employer's retirement account to capture the full match.

If your employer matches 50% of contributions up to 6% of your salary:
— On a $75,000 salary, 6% = $4,500 per year in your contributions
— Your employer adds $2,250 — free, immediate, guaranteed
— Failing to contribute that 6% means leaving $2,250 on the table every year

> — Over a 20-year career, that uncaptured match — compounded — could exceed $90,000
>
> Check your contribution rate today. If it is below the match threshold, change it this week. This is the single highest-return financial action most nurses can take immediately.

403(b) vs. 401(k) — What Nurses Need to Know

If you work at a nonprofit hospital, health system, or qualifying healthcare organization, your employer-sponsored retirement account is likely a 403(b). If you work at a for-profit system, it is likely a 401(k). For most practical purposes, they function identically — both allow pre-tax contributions that reduce your taxable income today, both grow tax-deferred, and both are taxed as ordinary income when you withdraw in retirement.

The contribution limits are the same: in 2024, you can contribute up to $23,000 per year (with an additional $7,500 catch-up contribution if you are fifty or older). The key difference for nurses working in nonprofit settings is that 403(b) participants may have access to an additional catch-up provision after fifteen years of service with the same employer — a benefit worth investigating with your HR department if you have tenure.

Account Type	Who It's For	Key Feature
403(b)	Nonprofit hospital/health system employees	15-year catch-up provision available; PSLF eligible employers
401(k)	For-profit health system employees	Standard pre-tax or Roth contribution options
Traditional IRA	Anyone with earned income	Tax deduction on contributions; taxed on withdrawal
Roth IRA	Income-eligible individuals	No tax deduction now; tax-FREE withdrawal in retirement
HSA	High-deductible health plan enrollees	Triple tax advantage — the most tax-efficient account that exists

The Roth IRA: The Account Every Nurse Should Know

If you are eligible — and many nurses are, depending on income — a Roth IRA is one of the most powerful wealth-building accounts available to an individual investor. You contribute after-tax dollars, which means you get no tax deduction today. In exchange, every dollar that the account grows — every dividend, every capital gain, every compounded return over the decades — is tax-free when you withdraw it in retirement.

For a nurse currently in a lower- or mid-range tax bracket who expects her income and tax rate to be higher later in her career, the Roth is a compelling choice. You pay tax on the seed rather than the harvest. For someone whose investment could grow significantly over twenty to thirty years, the tax-free harvest is an extraordinary advantage.

The contribution limit is $7,000 per year in 2024, with a $1,000 catch-up for those fifty and older. Income limits apply—check current IRS guidelines. But if you are eligible, maximizing your Roth IRA after claiming your employer match is one of the most strategic financial moves you can make.

Stocks: What They Are and Why They Matter

A stock is ownership. When you purchase a share of a company's stock, you own a small piece of that company — its assets, its future earnings, and its growth. If the company's value grows, your ownership stake grows with it. If it pays dividends, you receive a portion of its profits. If it declines, your stake declines as well.

Individual stock selection — choosing specific companies you believe will outperform — is a skill that takes years to develop, and most individual investors, including most financial professionals, do not consistently outperform the market average. This is not discouraging. It is liberating. Because there is an alternative that requires no stock-picking skill, minimal active management, and has outperformed the majority of actively managed funds over most long-term periods: the index fund.

Index Funds: The Investor's Scrubs

An index fund is a collection of stocks that mirrors a market index — the S&P 500, for example, which tracks the 500 largest publicly traded companies in the United States. When you invest in an S&P 500 index fund, you own a tiny piece of all five hundred companies. When the overall market grows, your investment grows. When it contracts, your investment contracts. You are not trying to beat the market. You are participating in it.

Think of it this way: individual stock picking is like trying to identify, in advance, which specific nurses on a unit will be the top performers next year. Index fund investing is like hiring the whole unit and benefiting from their collective output. The latter is less exciting. It is also far more reliable over time.

For nurses beginning to invest, a simple portfolio of low-cost index funds — a total US market fund, an international fund, and a bond fund in proportions that match your timeline and risk tolerance — is a starting point that financial researchers and Nobel-winning economists have defended for decades. It is not glamorous. It works.

A Simple Starting Investment Framework for Nurses

STEP 1: Capture the full employer match in your 403(b) or 401(k) — always first

STEP 2: Open and contribute to a Roth IRA if income-eligible — up to the annual limit

STEP 3: Inside both accounts, select low-cost index funds (look for expense ratios below 0.20%)

STEP 4: Set contributions to automatic — same date every month, without a decision required

STEP 5: Do not check daily. Do not react to market news. Do not stop during downturns.

Review your allocation once a year. Adjust as your income, timeline, and goals evolve.

That is the entire strategy for a beginning investor. Boring is not a weakness here — it is the method.

The Truth About Retirement Accounts — And Their Limits

I want to say something directly that most financial advisors soften into abstraction: your 401(k) or 403(b), on its own, will likely not be enough.

This is not a reason to abandon it — it is a reason to understand its role correctly. Employer retirement accounts are one instrument in a portfolio of wealth-building strategies. They are a powerful instrument, particularly with the employer match and the tax advantages. But they carry limitations that every nurse should understand before assuming they are fully covered.

They are illiquid until retirement age. Withdrawing before fifty-nine and a half triggers a ten percent penalty plus ordinary income tax — costs that can absorb a significant portion of what you have built. They are subject to market volatility. And they are designed to replace income in retirement — not to generate wealth before it, not to provide financial flexibility in your forties, not to fund the business opportunity or the real estate investment that appears when you are still in the building phase of your career.

What Your 403(b) Cannot Do — And What You Need Instead

Cannot be accessed before age 59.5 without penalty (with few exceptions)

Cannot fund a down payment on an investment property in your forties

Cannot generate income that replaces your salary while you are still working

Cannot provide liquidity for a business opportunity or an emergency

Cannot protect you from a market crash at the exact moment you need to withdraw

What fills these gaps: taxable brokerage accounts, real estate, business income, HSAs, and the diversified investment portfolio that Chapter 7 begins to build.

Retirement accounts are the floor. They are not the ceiling. Build above them.

The nurses who retire with genuine financial freedom are not the ones who maxed their 403(b) and called it a plan. They are the ones who used the 403(b) as a foundation and built multiple income streams above it — rental income, business income, taxable investment accounts, and other assets that do not require them to wait until they are 60 to access what they have built. That diversified approach is the subject of the next several chapters. But it begins here, with the understanding that the retirement account is a starting point, not a destination.

> ***Max your employer match. Open your Roth. Invest in index funds. And then — keep building. The retirement account is the floor. You deserve a house.***

Invest Wisely — What That Actually Means

'Invest wisely' is advice that sounds obvious until you try to follow it, at which point it becomes clear that nobody has defined what wisdom looks like in practice. Let me define it here, specifically for the nurse who is beginning.

Wise investing means understanding before you commit.

Do not put money into anything you cannot explain in two sentences. Not to a financial advisor. Not to a friend. To yourself. If you cannot explain what it is, how it makes money, what the risk is, and why you chose it, you do not understand it well enough to invest in it. This rule eliminates most bad investments before they happen. Cryptocurrency schemes, multilevel network investment opportunities, the hot stock tip from a colleague, the fund with extraordinary returns, and an explanation you could not quite follow — none of these pass the two-sentence test. Walk away.

Wise investing means diversification, not concentration.

Putting all your investment capital into one company, sector, asset class, or geographic market is not bold investing. It is risk concentration. The antidote is diversification — spreading your investment across asset types, markets, and time horizons so that the failure of any single component does not devastate the whole. Index funds are diversification made easy. A portfolio that includes equities, bonds, real estate, and cash equivalents is complete diversification.

Wise investing means matching your timeline to your strategy.

Money you will need in five years or less should not be in the stock market. Market volatility is real, and a correction at the wrong moment — right before you need to access the funds — can turn a disciplined investment into a costly loss. Money with a long timeline — twenty, thirty years — can absorb volatility and benefit from recovery. Know what each pool of money is for and invest it accordingly.

Wise investing means ignoring the noise.

The financial media, the market commentary, the quarterly performance anxiety — almost none of it is relevant to a nurse building long-term wealth through consistent, diversified investing. The markets will rise. The markets will fall. Both are temporary conditions. The investors who make the most money over time are not the ones who respond to the news most quickly. They are the ones who set a strategy, automated it, and had the discipline to leave it alone.

WISE INVESTING LOOKS LIKE	UNWISE INVESTING LOOKS LIKE
Starting small and consistently	Waiting until you have a large sum
Low-cost index funds	High-fee actively managed funds
Automatic monthly contributions	Investing only when you remember
Diversified portfolio	All-in on one stock or sector
Long-term horizon, ignoring noise	Reacting to market news and headlines
Understanding what you own	Investing in things you cannot explain
Employer match captured in full	Contributing below the match threshold
Building multiple income streams	Relying solely on the retirement account

The Nurse Who Invests Is Different — And She Knows It

There is something that shifts when you make your first investment. Not the investment itself — the shift happens in you. In the way you understand your relationship to money, to your income, to your future. You stop being someone to whom financial life happens and start being someone who directs it. The investment may be small. The shift is not.

I remember the first time I looked at a retirement account statement and understood what I was looking at — really understood it, not just the balance but the compounding trajectory, the projected value, the quiet work the money was doing without requiring any hours from me. That understanding changed how I thought about every shift I worked after that. Not because the work mattered less. But because the work's purpose had expanded. I was not just earning to spend. I was earning to build. And building, unlike earning, does not stop when you clock out.

The nurses in your unit who are quietly building wealth are probably not the ones with the most expensive cars in the parking lot. They are the ones who automate their contributions on payday and do not think about it again until the annual review. They are the ones who asked HR about the match in their first month of employment. They are the ones who started with what they had rather than waiting for the perfect amount. They look exactly like everyone else. Their balance sheets do not.

> ***The nurse who invests is not extraordinary. She is intentional. And intentionality, applied consistently over time, produces extraordinary outcomes.***

BOARDROOM MOMENT

Heal Your Wealth — Chapter 6 Reflection

Investing is not complicated once you remove the intimidation. Answer these questions and take one concrete action before you move to Chapter 7.

1. Log in to your employer benefits portal this week. What is your current retirement contribution rate? What is your employer's match — and are you contributing enough to capture it in full? If not, increase your contribution rate before the end of this month. This is the assignment.
2. Do you have a Roth IRA? If not, research eligibility based on your current income and open one if you qualify. If you already have one, are you contributing to it consistently? What would you need to adjust to reach the annual limit?
3. Look at the investments inside your 403(b) or 401(k). What are the expense ratios on the funds you are in? If any exceed 0.50%, research whether a lower-cost index fund alternative is available in your plan. Small differences in fees compound significantly over decades.
4. Write down every investment account you currently hold and its approximate balance. Now identify the gap: what is missing from this picture that Chapter 7 (real estate), Chapter 8 (entrepreneurship), or future chapters will begin to address? Name the next layer you want to build.
5. What is one thing you believed about investing before reading this chapter that you now understand differently? Write it down. The shift in understanding is the beginning of the shift in results.

Start small. Start now. The best investment you will ever make is the one you actually begin.

— — —

In Chapter 7, we move beyond the accounts your employer provides and into the investments you build yourself. Real estate — the asset class that has created more wealth for middle-income professionals than perhaps any other — demystified for the clinician who cannot attend a 9-to-5 closing, who works rotating shifts, and who may be starting from a smaller down payment than the standard advice assumes.

The property that generates income while you sleep is not reserved for people with more money than you. It is reserved for people with more information — and after this chapter, that is exactly what you are.

Continue to Chapter 7: Real Estate for the Working Clinician

CHAPTER SEVEN

Real Estate for the Working Clinician

On buying a home, building a legacy, and using property to set the pace for the generation that follows

I remember the first time I stood in a house I was considering buying and felt something shift in my chest.

It was not a grand house. It was not in a prestigious neighborhood. By the standards of what I had imagined for myself during the years of two jobs, tight budgets, and borrowed energy, it was modest. But it had a yard. It had a school district with good ratings on my internet search results. It had a street where children played in the afternoons and neighbors spoke to each other — the kind of environment I had been picturing in the abstract for years, but had never been close enough to touch.

I stood in the kitchen, and I thought: this is where my children will grow up. This is the neighborhood that will shape their early understanding of what is normal, what is safe, and what is possible. This is the address that will appear on their school applications, in their childhood photographs, and in the stories they tell their own children someday about where they came from.

That thought changed the way I understood real estate entirely. It was no longer a financial transaction. It was a declaration. A statement about the life I was choosing to build — not just for myself, but for the people I was building it for. And declarations, unlike rent payments, belong to you permanently.

> ***Buying a home is not just a financial decision. It is a declaration of belonging — to a neighborhood, to a future, to the generation that will carry what you build forward.***

The Neighborhood Is Not a Footnote

In most conversations about home buying, the neighborhood is treated as a preference — something you factor in alongside school ratings, commute time, and the square footage of the primary bedroom. I want to reframe it entirely: the neighborhood is the investment.

The house is a structure. Structures can be renovated, expanded, updated, and resold. The neighborhood — its safety, its social fabric, its school quality, the peer environment your children will grow up inside, the mental model they develop of what ordinary life looks like — cannot be renovated from within a single home. It is the context in which your family will live, and it shapes outcomes in ways that are difficult to overstate and impossible to separate from the property's financial return.

This is not an argument for spending beyond your means to live in the most expensive zip code available. It is an argument for treating neighborhood selection as a primary variable, not a secondary one — and for understanding that the school district, safety data, walkability, and the trajectory of local development are not quality-of-life considerations that sit alongside the financial analysis. They are part of it.

A home in a safe, improving neighborhood with strong schools will appreciate differently than the same-priced home in a neighborhood on a different trajectory. The equity you build is not only a function of the property — it is a function of everything around it. Choose the context deliberately.

What to Research Before Committing to a Neighborhood

School district ratings and trend direction — are they improving or declining over the past 5 years?

Crime statistics — look at trend data, not just current snapshots

Proximity to your workplace — commute time directly affects quality of life and fuel cost

Local development plans — new infrastructure, commercial investment, and zoning changes signal appreciation

Walkability and amenities — parks, grocery stores, community centers matter for family life and resale

Homeownership rate in the area — high ownership rates correlate with neighborhood stability

Property tax trajectory — rising taxes without corresponding service improvements erode your return

The neighborhood you choose will shape your children's lives and your property's value simultaneously.

Give it the research it deserves.

Legacy Begins With an Address

There is a difference between living somewhere and belonging somewhere. Renters, through no fault of their own, often live in the first condition. Homeowners have the genuine possibility — not the guarantee — of the second.

Belonging to a neighborhood means your children have consistent friendships rather than friendships that reset every time the lease terms shift. It means you have invested enough in a place to care about its school board elections, local infrastructure, and how its parks are maintained. It means the address on your mail is not a placeholder until the next move, but a coordinate from which you are building something permanent.

For immigrant healthcare professionals — for nurses and physicians and therapists who left countries where they had deep roots and crossed into a new place where they were starting from zero — the question of belonging carries particular weight. Owning a home in a neighborhood you chose deliberately, for reasons that reflect your values and your vision for your family, is an act of planting. You are saying: This is where we grow from here. This is the soil we are choosing.

That act — the choosing, the deliberate planting — reverberates forward in ways that are difficult to quantify but impossible to miss in the lives of children who grew up in homes their parents owned. The stability. The sense of permanence. The understanding, absorbed through daily life rather than any explicit teaching, that it is possible to build something that lasts.

What a Home Gives Your Children That Rent Cannot

A consistent neighborhood — the same friends, the same school, the same streets across the years that matter most.

A model of ownership — the living proof, experienced daily, that people like us build things that last.

Equity in their inheritance — the asset that may fund their education, their first home, their first business.

A sense of permanence — the deep psychological security of knowing that home is not contingent on a landlord's decision.

The story of how it started — the house where everything began, which they will tell their own children someday.

How Healthcare Professionals Are Uniquely Positioned to Buy

Healthcare professionals — nurses, physicians, advanced practice providers, therapists, pharmacists, and allied health clinicians — occupy an unusually strong position in the real estate market, and most of them do not fully know it.

The combination of stable, verifiable income, strong employment rates even in economic downturns, and the essential nature of healthcare work makes clinicians among the most creditworthy borrowers in any lending environment. Healthcare unemployment rates remain consistently lower than national averages across economic cycles. Lenders understand this. Real estate agents understand this. The question is whether you understand it—and whether you are positioning yourself to use it.

Loan Programs Designed for Healthcare Professionals

Several mortgage products exist specifically for or are particularly well-suited to healthcare professionals, and they deserve your attention before you assume you need a traditional twenty percent down payment to buy.

Loan Program	Who Qualifies	Key Advantage
Doctor / Clinician Loan	MDs, DOs, NPs, PAs, dentists, pharmacists, and some RNs	0–10% down, no PMI, student loans excluded or income-based in DTI calculation
FHA Loan	Any borrower with a 580+ credit score	3.5% down payment; accessible with moderate credit history
VA Loan	Veterans and active military (including many healthcare professionals)	0% down, no PMI, competitive rates — the most powerful loan program available
USDA Loan	Buyers in eligible rural/suburban areas	0% down for qualifying areas; many hospital-adjacent communities qualify
Conventional 97	First-time buyers with strong credit	3% down; lower total cost than FHA for borrowers with good credit
State First-Time Buyer Programs	Varies by state	Down payment assistance, grants, and reduced-rate programs — research your state's HFA

The physician or clinician loan program deserves particular attention from advanced practice providers and nurses in clinical leadership roles. These products were originally designed for physicians whose student debt-to-income ratios would otherwise disqualify them from conventional financing, and many have since expanded to include NPs, PAs, pharmacists, and, in some cases, RNs. The core advantage — the exclusion or income-based treatment of student loans in the debt-to-income calculation — can be the difference between qualifying for a home in the neighborhood you want and being pushed to a less desirable market.

Before you assume what you can afford, speak with a mortgage professional who has experience with healthcare professionals. The lending landscape available to you may be significantly different from the one described in general first-time buyer guides.

Your Credit Score Is the Price of Entry — Protect It

Every loan program, every interest rate, every mortgage product available to you is filtered through your credit score. The difference between a credit score of 680 and 760 on a 30-year mortgage can translate into tens of thousands of dollars in total interest paid over the life of the loan. That gap — paid in interest to a lender — is money that will not go toward your children's education, your retirement account, or your next investment property.

Protecting your credit score in the years before a home purchase means paying every bill on time without exception, keeping credit card utilization below thirty percent, avoiding new credit applications in the twelve months before you apply for a mortgage, and disputing any inaccuracies on your credit report as soon as they appear. These are not complicated actions. They are consistent ones.

The True Cost of Homeownership — Running the Honest Numbers

One of the most common mistakes first-time homebuyers make — including financially sophisticated healthcare professionals — is evaluating a home purchase based solely on the monthly mortgage payment. The mortgage payment is one line item. Homeownership has many.

The Complete Monthly Cost of Homeownership

Principal and interest (mortgage payment): $__________

Property taxes (annual amount divided by 12): $__________

Homeowner's insurance: $__________

HOA fees (if applicable): $__________

Private mortgage insurance / PMI (if applicable): $__________

Utilities (typically higher than renting): $__________

Maintenance reserve (budget 1–2% of home value/yr): $__________

TOTAL TRUE MONTHLY COST: $__________

This number — not the mortgage payment alone — is what homeownership costs.

Build this into your budget before you fall in love with a specific property.

The mortgage you can afford and the home you can afford are not always the same thing.

The maintenance reserve deserves particular emphasis because it is the cost most new homeowners do not budget for until the first major repair. A home is a physical structure, and physical structures require ongoing investment. The roof, the HVAC system, the plumbing, the appliances — all of them have lifespans and replacement costs. Setting aside 1 to 2 percent of your home's value each year for maintenance and repairs is not pessimism. It is the financial equivalent of preventive care: far less expensive than emergency intervention.

Beyond Your Primary Home: Real Estate as a Wealth-Building Strategy

The home you live in is an asset. But it is a particular kind of asset — one that builds equity over time and provides stability and belonging, but does not generate cash flow while you live in it. The next level of real estate wealth-building, the level that begins to produce income independent of your labor hours, requires thinking beyond the primary residence.

This is not as remote or as complex as it may sound. Healthcare professionals — with stable income, strong credit profiles, and knowledge of local markets around hospital systems — are well-positioned to begin building a real estate portfolio. The strategies available range from accessible starting points to sophisticated approaches, and you do not need to begin at the most complex level. You need to begin.

House Hacking — The Beginner's Entry Point

House hacking is the practice of purchasing a multi-unit property — a duplex, triplex, or small apartment building — living in one unit and renting the others. The rental income from the other units offsets, and in some cases, entirely covers your mortgage payment. You build equity in a property, live at a reduced or zero housing cost, and begin to develop the landlord skills and knowledge base that support future investment.

For a nurse or clinician who is not yet ready to maintain a separate investment property while managing a primary residence, house hacking is the entry point that makes the most financial sense. You are managing tenants in the building where you live. The learning curve is real, but so is the proximity. And the financial advantage — living effectively for free or near-free while building equity — is one of the most powerful first moves available to a debt-conscious healthcare professional building intentionally.

The Investment Property — Building Income-Producing Assets

Once your primary residence is stable and your emergency fund is in place, the next real estate layer is the income-producing rental property. This is the model my sister Collet demonstrated before I fully understood what I was watching: a property purchased and rented to tenants whose monthly payments cover the mortgage, taxes, insurance, and maintenance — and ideally produce positive cash flow above those costs.

The goal of a rental property is not appreciation alone. It is cash flow — the monthly income that arrives regardless of how many shifts you worked that week. That income, compounded across multiple properties over the years, is how real estate creates the kind of wealth that does not require your continuous physical presence to sustain.

Healthcare professionals are particularly well-suited to building rental portfolios because their income stability makes refinancing and portfolio growth more accessible, and because hospital corridors are some of the most reliable rental markets in any region. Properties near major medical centers command consistent demand from traveling nurses, medical residents, and healthcare staff—a tenant pool that the clinician-investor understands better than almost any other buyer.

RENTAL PROPERTY STRATEGY	WHAT MAKES IT RELEVANT FOR CLINICIANS
Long-term residential rental	Stable, consistent income; suits clinicians who want passive income without active management
Short-term rental (Airbnb / VRBO)	Higher income potential; requires more active management or a property manager
Travel nurse housing	Premium rents to healthcare travelers; clinicians understand this market from the inside
Medical district proximity rentals	Permanent demand from residents, interns, and clinical staff near hospital systems

House hacking (duplex / small multi-family)	Ideal first investment; reduces living costs while building equity and landlord experience
REITs (Real Estate Investment Trusts)	Stock-like real estate exposure; no property management; accessible with any investment amount

REITs — Real Estate Without the Landlord Responsibilities

Not every healthcare professional has the bandwidth to manage a rental property — and the honest answer is that direct property ownership is not the right strategy for every season of a clinician's life. For those who want real estate exposure in their investment portfolio without the operational complexity of property ownership, Real Estate Investment Trusts offer a compelling alternative.

A REIT is a company that owns, operates, or finances income-producing real estate. When you purchase shares of a REIT, you are effectively owning a fraction of a large real estate portfolio — office buildings, apartment complexes, healthcare facilities, warehouses — without the responsibilities of a landlord. REITs are required by law to distribute at least 90% of their taxable income to shareholders as dividends, making them a reliable source of passive income in an investment portfolio.

Healthcare REITs, in particular, are a category that clinicians may find both familiar and compelling: these funds own hospitals, medical office buildings, senior living facilities, and other healthcare infrastructure assets whose demand is driven by the same demographic trends that are expanding the healthcare workforce. You understand this sector. That is a legitimate investment edge.

Real Estate Investment Options at Every Stage

STAGE 1 — Getting Started (primary home purchased, emergency fund in place):

→ House hack a duplex or small multi-family as your primary residence

→ Add REITs to your investment portfolio through your brokerage account

STAGE 2 — Building (primary home stable, debt eliminated or managed):

→ Purchase first standalone rental property near a hospital or medical center

→ Consider travel nurse short-term rental in a high-demand market

STAGE 3 — Scaling (multiple properties, professional management in place):

→ Refinance to pull equity from existing properties and fund new acquisitions

→ Explore commercial real estate or larger multi-family properties

→ Consider a self-directed IRA to hold real estate in a tax-advantaged account

You do not need to start at Stage 3. You need to start at Stage 1—and begin.

What Collet Built — And What It Taught Me

I have referenced my sister Collet throughout this book as the model of financial intentionality I did not yet have language for when I was watching her live it. Nowhere is that model more relevant than in this chapter.

Collet owned two properties. One was the home we shared — the stability she provided while I was finding my footing in a new country and a new career. The other was an investment property that generated monthly rental income, without her having to work an additional shift to produce it. She had built a second income stream not from extra hours but from an asset — and the difference between those two sources of income is the entire argument of this chapter.

Her overtime, when she worked it, went to a specific place. It funded the down payment, it serviced the investment, and it built the equity that eventually became options. She was not in the overtime trap because her lifestyle was not built around overtime. Her lifestyle was built around her baseline, and overtime built something above it.

That model — income-producing assets that work independently of your labor hours — is the goal that real estate enables healthcare professionals to achieve at almost every income level. You do not need to replicate it exactly. You need to understand the principle and start building your own version.

> ***An asset that generates income while you sleep is not a luxury reserved for the wealthy. It is the mechanism by which people become wealthy — and real estate is the most accessible version of it for the working clinician.***

Setting the Pace for the Generation That Follows

Here is the truth about generational wealth that nobody in your family's financial history may have told you: it does not begin with a large inheritance. It begins with a decision. A single decision, made by one person in one generation, that changes the starting point for everyone who comes after.

The home you buy in a safe neighborhood sets a starting point for your children that is categorically different from the one you had. Not because the house is grand — it does not have to be grand because it is owned. Because equity builds rather than rent disappears. Because when your children watch you make mortgage payments, they are watching you build something that belongs to your family rather than your landlord. Because when they leave for college or for their first job or for their first apartment, they leave from a home — not from a rental unit, but from a home — and that difference leaves a mark that is impossible to fully articulate and impossible to overestimate fully.

You are not just buying property. You are setting the pace. You are establishing the baseline expectation for what is normal, what is achievable, and what people in your family build. Your children will not remember the sacrifice that made the down payment possible. They will remember the yard, the neighborhood, the school, and the street. And they will carry that as their model of what home means — which is the most durable inheritance you can leave them.

What You Are Building When You Buy

For yourself: equity, stability, and the specific peace of knowing the roof is yours.

For your children: a model of ownership, a safe neighborhood, a school district chosen with intention.

For your family: the beginning of an asset portfolio that can be inherited, leveraged, and built upon.

For the generation that follows: a different starting point. A higher floor. A wider horizon.

You are not just buying a house. You are writing the first chapter of a different financial story for everyone who comes after you.

The Practical Path to Your First Home — A Checklist

The home purchase process is not complicated once it is demystified. Here is the sequence that applies to most first-time healthcare professional buyers, with the specific considerations relevant to clinicians highlighted at each stage.

Your Home Buying Roadmap — Healthcare Professional Edition

STEP 1: CLEAN THE FINANCIAL BASELINE

→ Net worth calculated and documented (Chapter 2)

→ Consumer debt eliminated or on active repayment plan (Chapter 3)

→ Budget built around baseline income — home purchase fits within it (Chapter 4)

→ Credit score pulled and reviewed — target 700+ before applying

STEP 2: BUILD THE DOWN PAYMENT AND RESERVE

→ Down payment saved (3–20% depending on loan program)

→ Closing costs reserved separately (typically 2–5% of purchase price)

→ Emergency fund intact after closing — do not drain savings to zero

→ First-year maintenance reserve identified (1–2% of purchase price)

STEP 3: UNDERSTAND YOUR FINANCING OPTIONS

→ Research clinician loan programs available in your state

→ Get pre-approved with two or three lenders to compare rates

→ Understand what your student loans mean for your DTI calculation

→ Investigate state down payment assistance programs

STEP 4: SELECT STRATEGICALLY
→ Neighborhood research completed — school, safety, trajectory
→ Total monthly cost calculated — mortgage plus all associated costs
→ Resale potential assessed — is this a neighborhood people are moving toward?
→ Long-term fit evaluated — does this home serve your family for 5–10+ years?

STEP 5: CLOSE WITH CONFIDENCE
→ Home inspection completed — do not skip this
→ Title insurance in place
→ All documents reviewed before signing — understand what you are signing
→ Celebrate. You have built something permanent.

BOARDROOM MOMENT

Heal Your Wealth — Chapter 7 Reflection

Real estate is the asset class most associated with generational wealth — and the most available to healthcare professionals at any income level, if approached with the right information and the right strategy.

6. If you do not yet own a home: what is the specific gap between where you are today and where you need to be to qualify? Name it precisely — credit score, down payment, debt-to-income ratio. That gap is your assignment, not your obstacle.
7. Research clinician or professional loan programs available in your state this week. Call or email two lenders with experience in healthcare professional lending. Ask them specifically what programs you qualify for and what they require. Write down what you learn.
8. Describe the neighborhood you want your children to grow up in — not abstractly, but specifically. School rating, commute distance to your workplace, the feel of the street, and the community you want to belong to. Now, research what that neighborhood costs and what the path from here to there looks like.
9. If you already own your primary residence, have you considered the next layer? Research one investment property strategy from this chapter — house hacking, a rental near a medical center, or a healthcare REIT. What would it take to make that your next financial move?
10. Write the legacy sentence: 'The home I am building toward will give my children ____________.' Complete it with something specific—not a dollar amount, but a life condition. Safety. Stability. A school where they thrive. A neighborhood that expands

what they believe is possible for people like them. That sentence is your real estate strategy's north star.

The home you buy is not just an address. It is a declaration of permanence, of intention, of the life you are building on purpose. Make the declaration wisely.

— — —

In Chapter 8, we turn to the entrepreneurial instinct that lives in almost every healthcare professional who has ever thought, "There is a better way to do this." The business idea, the clinical consulting practice, the healthcare venture that serves a need you identified from within the profession. Building income that does not depend on a single employer or a single shift — and doing it without losing the clinical foundation that makes you credible.

The entrepreneur nurse is not a departure from the clinician. She is the fullest expression of one.

Continue to Chapter 8: The Entrepreneur Clinician

CHAPTER EIGHT

The Entrepreneur Clinician

Be curious. Learn. Explore. The healthcare profession fits everywhere — and so do you.

A lot of people graduate from nursing school, get their first med-surg job, and become content.

I say this not as a criticism — med-surg is where clinical foundations are built, where the work is real, the stakes are immediate, and the learning is relentless. There is dignity in that work. There is value in that work. But there is a version of the content that is actually comfortable, and another that is simply unexplored. And too many healthcare professionals spend their careers in the second kind without ever discovering how much farther the first kind could have taken them.

The nursing profession is one of the most adaptable credentials in existence. It goes everywhere. It fits inside hospitals and clinics and schools and courtrooms and boardrooms and research institutions and policy chambers and startup companies and international aid organizations and technology firms that need clinical expertise to build products that actually serve patients. The scope of what a healthcare professional can do with their training — once they become curious enough to look — is staggering. And most of them never look. Not because the opportunities are hidden, but because the first job was available and the comfort of the familiar is a powerful sedative.

This chapter is the antidote to that sedation. It is an invitation to look up from the unit and ask: what else is this credential capable of? What else am I capable of? And then — more importantly — to go find out.

> ***You did not spend years earning this credential to park it at the first available exit. Healthcare is vast. Your potential inside it is broader than any single job title.***

The Danger of Comfortable

Let me describe comfortable, so you know it when you see it in yourself.

Comfortable is the nurse who has been on the same unit for eight years and knows exactly where everything is, exactly how the charge nurse schedules, exactly which physicians are easy to work with and which are not. She is competent, reliable, and valued. She has also not attended a conference in three years, has not read a clinical journal in longer than that, and has not seriously asked herself what else might be possible since the first year she stopped feeling like a beginner.

Comfortable is the physician assistant who took the first permanent position offered after graduation and has been there for six years, not because it is the best fit, but because the process of looking for something better requires energy that the current job has been steadily consuming. She tells herself she will explore her options when things slow down. Things have not slowed down. They will not.

Comfortable is the clinical pharmacist who knows her role thoroughly and executes it well, but who has never investigated what her credentials make possible outside the dispensary — in medication therapy management, clinical research, pharmaceutical consulting, and healthcare technology. Not because she lacks curiosity, but because the job provided the structure that made curiosity feel unnecessary.

None of these people is a failure. They are simply unexplored. And unexplored potential in a profession as broad as healthcare is one of the most expensive forms of financial loss a clinician can sustain — because the income that was available but not pursued cannot be recovered. The years in which the credential could have compounded in value were instead spent at a static level.

> ***Comfortable is not the same as fulfilled. And fulfilled is not the same as maximized. The profession is too broad and your career too short to confuse any of the three.***

Where Healthcare Professionals Actually Work

Most healthcare professionals have a mental map of their profession that is far smaller than the territory. The mental map includes the hospital, the clinic, and the long-term care facility — the places where clinical training prepared them and where the majority of their peers can be found. The territory is considerably larger.

Where Your Healthcare Credential Can Take You — Beyond the Bedside

CLINICAL LEADERSHIP & ADMINISTRATION

Director of Clinical Operations, Chief Nursing Officer, VP of Patient Services, Chief Medical Officer, Department Chair, Quality and Compliance Director

ENTREPRENEURSHIP & BUSINESS

Independent NP / PA practice owner, clinical staffing agency founder, healthcare consulting firm, medical supply, and pharmaceutical distribution, home health agency, occupational health consulting

TECHNOLOGY & INNOVATION

Clinical informaticist, health tech startup advisor, EHR implementation consultant, telehealth clinical director, medical device clinical specialist, AI health product reviewer

EDUCATION & ACADEMIA

Clinical faculty, simulation lab director, nursing school professor, continuing education content developer, clinical preceptor program director

RESEARCH & POLICY

Clinical research coordinator, principal investigator, sub-investigator, healthcare policy analyst, government health agency consultant, WHO, and NGO roles

MEDIA, CONTENT & THOUGHT LEADERSHIP

Healthcare author, podcast host, keynote speaker, clinical content creator, medical expert witness, healthcare journalist, brand ambassador for clinical products

GLOBAL HEALTH

International health program director, medical mission leadership, pharmaceutical distribution in emerging markets, global health consulting

I have personally occupied several of these roles simultaneously. As a board-certified Family Nurse Practitioner, I have managed clinical teams across four states. As Director of Clinical Operations, I have led systems and people at an executive level. As a sub-investigator in clinical research, I have contributed to the evidence base that shapes how medicine is practiced. As co-founder of Icon Oncology Supply, I have built a pharmaceutical distribution company operating across East Africa. As host of the Money Moves Daily podcast, I have built a platform that teaches financial literacy to thousands of healthcare professionals.

None of these roles was available to me on the day I graduated from nursing school. All of them became available when I refused to accept that the first job was the full map.

What 'I Refuse to Settle' Actually Built

Managing clinicians across four states as an NP — because I asked what multi-state practice looked like.

Director of Clinical Operations — because I pursued executive leadership, not just clinical excellence.

Sub-investigator in clinical research — because I said yes to the opportunity before I felt fully ready.

Co-founder of a pharmaceutical company operating in Kenya — because I saw a need and trusted my training to meet it.

Author. Podcast host. Executive. Entrepreneur.

All of it grew from one refusal: the refusal to let the first available option define the ceiling.

Curiosity Is a Career Strategy

In clinical training, curiosity is treated as a diagnostic virtue — the clinician who keeps asking why, who does not accept a presentation at face value, who follows the question past the obvious answer to the real one, is the clinician who finds what others miss. That same intellectual disposition, applied to your career rather than your patient panel, is one of the most powerful professional development strategies available to a healthcare professional.

Curiosity means attending conferences not to collect continuing education credits but to encounter ideas you did not know existed. It means reading outside your specialty — healthcare technology, healthcare policy, global health, financial strategy — to understand the landscape in which your clinical skills operate. It means having conversations with people in adjacent roles and asking not what do you do but how did you get there and what did you wish you had known. It means treating your career the way you were trained to treat a patient: with systematic inquiry, ongoing assessment, and a willingness to update the plan when new information arrives.

The healthcare professionals who build the most interesting, most financially rewarding, and most fulfilling careers are not always the ones with the most impressive credentials at graduation. They are the ones who stayed curious after graduation. Who kept asking. Who kept looking. Who treated the credential not as a destination but as a platform—and kept building on it.

The Curiosity Habit — Five Practices That Expand Your Career Horizon

1. Read one article or paper per week outside your immediate specialty or role.
   Healthcare tech, policy, global health, business — pick a direction and rotate quarterly.

2. Attend at least one conference or professional event per year that is not your unit's routine.
   The room where ideas are exchanged is the room where opportunities are born.

3. Follow three to five healthcare professionals on LinkedIn whose career paths you find interesting.
   Not to imitate them — to see what is possible in directions you had not considered.

4. Ask one 'what else' question every quarter: What else could this credential do? What else is happening in this specialty? What else am I not seeing from where I currently stand?

5. Say yes to one opportunity that feels slightly beyond your current comfort level per year. The committee seat, the presentation, the pilot program, the unfamiliar assignment. Growth lives exactly one step past comfortable.

Certifications: The Currency of Clinical Advancement

If curiosity is the disposition, certifications are often the mechanism. In healthcare, a certification is not merely a credential to display on a badge — it is a signal to employers, patients, and colleagues that you have invested in a specific depth of knowledge, that you meet a recognized standard, and that you take your professional development seriously enough to pursue it on your own time and your own terms.

More concretely, certifications translate directly into earning power. Specialty certifications in emergency nursing, critical care, oncology, informatics, diabetes education, wound care, infection control, and dozens of other areas command premium rates in both clinical and consulting contexts. The investment in the certification — the study time, the examination fee, the continuing education to maintain it — is almost always recovered in the income differential it creates, often within a single year.

Certification	Field	Career Impact
FNP-BC / AGPCNP-BC	Nurse Practitioner Practice	Multi-state practice authority, independent prescribing, and leadership roles
CCRN	Critical Care Nursing	Premium pay in ICU, CVICU, MICU; leadership and transport roles
CEN	Emergency Nursing	ED charge positions, flight nursing, trauma center roles
OCN	Oncology Nursing	Specialty oncology roles, research, and pharmaceutical consulting
CDCES	Diabetes Care & Education	Independent practice, consulting, corporate wellness programs
CPHRM	Healthcare Risk Management	Hospital administration, insurance, and legal consulting

CPHQ	Healthcare Quality	Quality director roles, accreditation consulting, and regulatory affairs
ACHE Fellowship (FACHE)	Healthcare Executive Leadership	C-suite credibility, board eligibility, and executive compensation
CRC	Clinical Research	Site coordinator, sub-investigator, CRO consulting
RHIA / RHIT	Health Information Management	Informatics, EHR consulting, technology roles

The principle is not to accumulate certifications indiscriminately — each one requires investment of time and money that should be weighed against the return it generates in your specific career trajectory. The principle is to treat certifications as strategic investments: ask what doors this credential opens, what income differential it creates, and whether the roles it enables align with the career you are intentionally building. If the answer is yes on all three, pursue it with focus.

Conferences and Seminars: The Rooms That Change Careers

I want to make an argument for conferences that goes beyond continuing education credits — because credits are the least valuable thing a conference offers.

The most valuable thing a conference offers is the room. The physical or virtual space where people who are doing interesting things in your field have gathered, where conversations happen between scheduled sessions, where the person sitting next to you at lunch turns out to be building exactly the kind of organization you have been thinking about, where the keynote speaker describes a career path you did not know existed and you write down everything she says.

I have attended conferences that changed the direction of my career. Not because of the formal curriculum — though that mattered — but because of who was in the room and what became possible when I was in it with them. The introduction that led to a collaboration. The panel discussion that framed a problem I had been carrying, but couldn't name. The conversation in the exhibitor hall turned into a consulting opportunity. The colleague I met who became a mentor. None of these appear on the continuing education transcript. All of them shaped the trajectory.

High-Value Conferences for Healthcare Professionals at Every Stage

NURSING & ADVANCED PRACTICE

AANP National Conference (NPs) | NAPNAP (Pediatric NPs) | ONS Congress (Oncology)

ANA National Nursing Conference | AONE / AONL (Nursing Leadership)

HEALTHCARE LEADERSHIP & EXECUTIVE

ACHE Congress on Healthcare Leadership | Becker's Hospital Review Conference
HIMSS (Health Information & Management) | IHI National Forum (Quality & Safety)

CLINICAL SPECIALTIES

ACEP Scientific Assembly (Emergency) | SCCM Critical Care Congress
ASH Annual Meeting (Hematology) | ASCO Annual Meeting (Oncology)

ENTREPRENEURSHIP & INNOVATION

Rock Health Summit | Health 2.0 | StartUp Health Festival
Black Healthcare Leaders Conference | National Black Nurses Association Conference

RESEARCH

ACRP Annual Conference (Clinical Research) | APHA Annual Meeting

Rule: Attend one outside your immediate specialty per year.
The most valuable room is the one where you are the only person who does what you do.

The New Trends Every Healthcare Professional Should Know

The healthcare landscape is changing at a pace that rewards the curious and disadvantages the static. The clinician who understands what is happening at the edges of the profession — the technological shifts, the regulatory changes, the emerging practice models — is not just better informed. She is better positioned. Better positioned for the roles that are being created, for the consulting opportunities that are expanding, for the entrepreneurial gaps that are opening as the industry reshapes itself.

Telehealth and Multi-State Practice

The expansion of telehealth — accelerated by the pandemic and now embedded in the permanent fabric of healthcare delivery — has transformed the geographic reality of clinical practice. Nurse practitioners and physicians who hold licensure in multiple states can now build clinical practices that are not constrained by the radius of a single hospital system or the commute to a single clinic. Multi-state practice through the Nurse Licensure Compact, combined with telehealth platforms, means that a clinician with the right credentials and infrastructure can serve patients across a region — or even a country — from a single location.

I manage clinical teams across four states. That was not possible at the beginning of my career in the way it is now. The infrastructure for it — the regulatory framework, the technology, the reimbursement models — has matured. The clinician who understands how to operate within it, build a multi-state practice, and leverage telehealth as a business platform rather than simply a clinical convenience is positioned for a category of earnings and impact that did not exist a decade ago.

Clinical Research — The Credential That Compounds

Clinical research is one of the most underutilized career pathways in nursing and allied health, and one of the most financially rewarding for clinicians who pursue it with intention. Research coordinators, sub-investigators, and principal investigators are in consistent demand at academic medical centers, pharmaceutical companies, contract research organizations, and independent site networks. The skills are learnable, the credential is obtainable, and the income premium over standard clinical roles is significant.

Beyond income, clinical research experience builds a professional profile that opens doors to pharmaceutical consulting, medical affairs roles, and regulatory advisory positions — all of which compensate at levels well above standard clinical practice. For the clinician who is curious about how medicine is made — how treatments are developed, how evidence is built — this pathway deserves serious investigation.

Healthcare Entrepreneurship and Business Building

The clinician who identifies a problem from inside the system and builds a solution to it has an advantage that no MBA can replicate: she understands the problem in her body, not just in a case study. The most compelling healthcare businesses are almost always founded by people who experienced the gap they are trying to close — who were the patient, the nurse, the physician who kept hitting the same wall and eventually decided to build a door.

Entrepreneurial opportunities available to healthcare professionals include independent clinical practice, staffing and workforce solutions, home health and private duty care, medical education and training, health coaching and wellness, pharmaceutical and medical supply distribution, clinical consulting, and healthcare technology advisory. The common thread is clinical expertise applied to a business context, a combination the market consistently underserves and consistently rewards.

Health Technology and Informatics

Every electronic health record system, every patient monitoring platform, every clinical decision support tool, every telehealth application requires clinical input to be useful rather than merely functional. The healthcare technology industry is hungry for clinicians who understand both the clinical workflow and the technological landscape — who can translate between engineers and bedside nurses, and who can assess whether a product actually serves the patient encounter it claims to support.

Clinical informatics, health IT consulting, and technology advisory roles are growing rapidly, compensate significantly above standard clinical rates, and are available to nurses and allied health professionals at all levels of technical sophistication. You do not need to be a programmer. You need to understand clinical workflow and be willing to learn the technological context that surrounds it.

Emerging Trend	What It Creates	How to Position Yourself
Telehealth expansion	Multi-state practice opportunities	Obtain compact licensure; build telehealth platform literacy
Clinical AI tools	Clinical AI advisor and reviewer roles	Learn AI fundamentals; join clinical AI working groups
Value-based care models	Quality and outcomes consulting	Study population health management; pursue CPHQ
Nursing workforce shortage	Staffing and workforce consulting	Build expertise in retention, staffing ratios, and workforce strategy
Global health expansion	International clinical leadership	Develop global health competencies; explore WHO and NGO networks
Mental health integration	Behavioral health consulting roles	Pursue a psychiatric NP or behavioral health certification
Retail and employer health	Direct primary care and employer clinics	Study direct care models; explore employer health contracting

Building Income Beyond the Salary

The entrepreneur-clinician does not think of income as a single stream. She thinks about income architecture — the deliberate design of multiple channels through which her clinical expertise generates revenue, not all of which require her physical presence at a clinical site on any given day.

The salary from the primary clinical role is the foundation. It is reliable, it provides benefits, and it maintains the clinical currency that makes everything else credible. But it is one stream. The entrepreneur clinician builds beside it, above it, and eventually, partly independent of it.

Income Streams Available to the Entrepreneur Clinician

PRIMARY INCOME (time-for-money, foundation):

Salary or hourly clinical role — the baseline that funds the building

ACTIVE SECONDARY INCOME (time-for-money, higher rate):

Consulting: clinical auditing, regulatory, quality, telehealth

Expert witness testimony for medical-legal cases

Per diem / locum tenens practice at premium rates

Clinical education: university adjunct faculty, simulation instruction
Speaking: conferences, corporate health events, community education

LEVERAGED INCOME (expertise once, income repeatedly):
Online course or certification program built on clinical expertise
Book or published work generating royalties
Podcast or digital content with sponsorship and affiliate income
Licensing clinical protocols or educational materials

PASSIVE INCOME (money working without your hours):
Rental property income (Chapter 7)
Investment portfolio dividends and appreciation (Chapter 6)
Business equity in a healthcare venture

The goal is not to build all of these at once.
The goal is to deliberately build one additional stream, then another, over time.
Each stream you add is one fewer shift you must take to sustain the life you are building.

You Will Be Surprised

I want to close this chapter with the sentence I have said to nurses, physicians, pharmacists, and therapists in every professional context I have occupied, because it is the truest thing I know about healthcare professionals and their unexplored potential:

You will be surprised.

You will be surprised by what your credentials make accessible when you stop assuming the first job was the full map. You will be surprised by the conversations that begin when you walk into a conference with curiosity rather than obligation. You will be surprised by the opportunities that appear when you start saying yes to things that feel slightly beyond you — because the stretch is where growth lives, and growth is where the income and the impact and the fulfillment are waiting.

I was surprised. I arrived in America as an IT professional and did not know that I would become a nurse. I became a nurse and did not know that I would become a nurse practitioner managing teams across four states. I became an NP and did not know that I would co-found a pharmaceutical company operating in East Africa. Each of those surprises was available to me because I refused to let the current chapter feel like the final one — and because I stayed curious enough to keep asking what else.

What else is your credential capable of? What else are you capable of? What else is available in the profession you have spent years earning the right to practice?

Go find out. Be curious. Learn. Explore.

And then come back and teach someone else what you found.

> ***The healthcare profession fits everywhere. So do you. The only question is how far you are willing to look — and how long you are willing to keep looking after comfortable stops feeling like enough.***

A Message to the Clinician Who Has Been Comfortable Long Enough

The unit needs you. And the world outside it also needs you.

The certification you have been putting off—start the application.

The conference you have been meaning to attend — register this month.

The idea you have been carrying for three years — write it down and take one step toward it.

The career you imagined before the first job made the imaginable feel impractical — it is still possible.

Go look for it. Intentionally. With everything you have already built as your foundation.

You will be surprised how far it takes you.

BOARDROOM MOMENT

Heal Your Wealth – Chapter 8 Reflection

Contentment is not a virtue when it costs you your potential. These questions are designed to surface the next version of your career — the one curiosity builds.

11. What is the most interesting role you have encountered in healthcare that is not your current one? What would it take — in credentials, in experience, in positioning — to move toward it? Map the gap between where you are and where that role begins.
12. When did you last attend a professional event — conference, seminar, webinar, or workshop — that was outside your immediate clinical unit or specialty? If the answer is more than a year ago, what is the next one you will attend, and when will you register for it?
13. List every certification you currently hold. Now, research one additional certification in your specialty or in an adjacent area that would expand your scope, increase your income, or open a door you cannot currently access. What is the certification, what does it require, and what is your target date to achieve it?

14. Describe one entrepreneurial opportunity you have identified from inside the healthcare system — a gap, a need, an inefficiency, a service that patients clearly need and that no one is providing well. You do not need a business plan yet. Just describe the opportunity in one paragraph.
15. Write the 'what else' sentence for your career right now: 'My credentials make possible something I have not yet pursued, which is ____________.' Complete it honestly. Then ask: what is the first step toward that thing, and when will I take it?

You did not cross every obstacle that brought you to this profession to stay exactly where you landed on day one. The profession is broad. Your potential is broader. Go find out how far it reaches.

— — —

In Chapter 9, we go deeper into the most personal territory in this book: the stories we tell about money, the performances we maintain to protect those stories, and what becomes possible when we finally take the mask off. The lies we portray and the reality we live — and the healing that begins when we decide to close the gap between them.

You have spent this chapter looking outward — at the breadth of the profession, the width of the opportunity, the distance between where you are and where the credential can take you. Chapter 9 turns the lens inward. Because no external opportunity will be fully accessible to a healthcare professional who is not honest with herself, first, about the financial and emotional reality she is actually living.

Continue to Chapter 9: The Lies We Portray, The Reality We Live

CHAPTER NINE

The Lies We Portray, The Reality We Live

Money, Identity & Culture — this is where the mask comes off, and healing begins

I want to tell you about a nurse I know.

She walks into the unit every morning looking put together. Her scrubs are pressed. Her shoes are clean. She laughs easily in the break room, talks about her weekend plans, and mentions something offhand about a dinner she went to. Her colleagues think of her as someone who has it together — someone who has figured out the balance between a demanding career and a full life. She is liked. She is respected. She carries herself with a quiet confidence that people notice.

She is also working seven days a week because she cannot afford not to.

Her credit cards are close to their limits. Her savings account holds less than one month of expenses. Overtime is not a choice — it hasn't been for a long time — but she has never said that out loud. To anyone. Because the gap between the version of herself she presents and the reality she returns to every evening is one she has been protecting for years, with enormous energy, at enormous cost.

I know her because in a significant season of my own career, I was her.

> ***We spend so much energy maintaining the appearance of financial stability that we have almost none left to actually build it.***

The Performance of Financial Wellness

There is a performance that many healthcare professionals put on — in the break room, on social media, in casual conversations with colleagues — about their financial lives. It is not malicious. It is not calculated deception. It is the entirely human response to a culture that equates financial struggle with personal failure, and that has never provided a safe space for nurses — who are expected to be capable, composed, and in control — to say out loud: "I am not doing as well as I look."

The performance looks like this: the casual mention of the vacation you are planning that you are actually going to put on a credit card. The silence when a colleague asks if you are going to the conference, because the registration fee is not in your budget, and you do not know how to say that. The extra shift you pick up on a Saturday, framed as a choice — I just wanted to get the hours in — when the truth is the rent autopays on Monday and the account isn't there yet.

It looks like exhaustion is explained away as dedication. Stress is explained away as busyness. A financial reality that bears almost no resemblance to the professional identity you have worked so hard to build and protect.

WHAT WE SAY	WHAT IT COSTS US
"I picked up an extra shift — I just wanted the hours."	The truth stays hidden. The cycle continues. The shame grows.
"I'm fine financially, just a bit busy right now."	We lose the chance to ask for help, mentorship, or community.
"I like to keep busy — the overtime keeps me sharp."	We normalize overwork instead of addressing its financial root.
"Things are great — just working hard toward my goals."	We perform wellness we do not feel, at the cost of real connection.
Silence when the conversation turns to savings or investing.	We stay isolated in our financial struggle, believing we are alone.

The performance is exhausting. And it is one of the most significant barriers to financial healing — because you cannot heal what you will not name, and you cannot name what you are committed to hiding.

Why We Do It — The Culture Behind the Mask

To understand why so many nurses maintain this performance, you have to understand the culture in which nurses are formed.

Nursing culture prizes resilience. It prizes the ability to absorb difficulty without visible strain — to manage the weight of what clinical work demands without bringing it into the break room, without letting it show on your face in front of patients, without admitting to anyone that today was harder than you had capacity for. This is a survival skill in a demanding profession. It is also, when applied to financial life, a trap.

The same trait that makes nurses exceptional caregivers — the capacity to appear composed while carrying significant strain — makes financial vulnerability nearly impossible to express. To say I am struggling financially in a nursing unit is to crack the composure that everyone has silently agreed is mandatory. And so nurses do not say it. They manage. They perform. They pick up another shift and keep the mask in place.

For many immigrant nurses, the pressure is compounded. You left home, crossed an ocean, sacrificed proximity to everything familiar in pursuit of a better life. Admitting financial struggle in that context can feel like admitting that the sacrifice was not worth it — that the promise of the journey has not been kept. And so the performance extends even to the family back home, who may not know the full picture of the immigrant nurse's American financial life.

> ***The culture that made you resilient also taught you to hide. Healing begins when you learn the difference between strength and silence.***

The Specific Lie About Overtime

Of all the financial performances nurses maintain, the one about overtime may be the most universal and the most damaging.

The lie is simple: I work extra shifts because I want to, not because I have to. It is delivered with confidence, sometimes with pride, and it is believed — by colleagues, by family, sometimes even by the nurse herself after she has repeated it enough times. The alternative — saying I work extra shifts because my budget requires it and I do not know how to close the gap any other way — feels like a confession of failure. And so the script stays clean. The overtime is framed as a choice. The necessity stays invisible.

But the necessity does not stay invisible to the body. The necessity does not go unnoticed by the family that sees the fatigue, hears the short answers at the end of seven days, and watches the nurse move through her days off in a fog of recovery rather than presence. The reality of what the overtime costs are is lived by everyone close to her, even when the story she tells remains the curated one.

And the cost of maintaining that story is profound. Because as long as overtime is framed as a choice, there is no urgency to address the financial structure that makes it necessary. The lie protects the status quo. And the status quo keeps the revolving door turning.

The Moment the Story Changes

The story changes the moment you say — even just to yourself, even just on paper — the truth:

"I am working extra shifts because my budget requires it."
"I am tired in ways that my days off cannot fully address."
"The overtime is not a choice. And I want it to become one."

That sentence — said honestly, without performance, to yourself — is the beginning.

Not the end of the struggle. The beginning of the healing.

Everything this book has taught you up to this point is the toolkit.

This is the moment you pick it up.

Identity and the Money Story

Your identity is inseparable from your money story. Not because money defines who you are — it does not, and this book has never argued that it does — but because the beliefs you carry about money were formed in the same crucible as everything else that makes you who you are: your family, your culture, your childhood, your immigration story, your professional formation, your accumulated experience of what happens when financial reality does not match financial aspiration.

For many nurses, the money story begins long before the first paycheck. It begins in a home where money was scarce and unspoken about — where its absence was felt but never examined, where its management was modeled as survival rather than strategy. It begins in a culture where financial struggle is normalized, where working multiple jobs is a badge of honor rather than a symptom of a system that needs redesigning, where saving and investing are concepts that belong to other people — people with more, people with different starting points, people whose story began in a different place than yours.

Those stories are not your fault. They were given to you before you had the capacity to question them. But they are yours now — and the question is whether you will continue to live inside them, or whether you will write something different.

> ***The money story you inherited is not a life sentence. It is a starting chapter. You are the author of everything that comes after.***

The Identity Shift That Changes Everything

The shift I am describing is not primarily financial. It is not a new budget, a new investment account, or a new debt-elimination strategy. All of those matter—we have spent eight chapters building them. But they sit on top of something deeper, and that deeper thing is this: you have to decide who you are in relation to money.

Not who your family was. Not who nursing culture tells you to be. Not the performance you have maintained in the break room or on social media. Who you actually are, and who you are choosing to become.

I am a woman who grew up watching paycheck-to-paycheck living modeled as the only option. I am an immigrant who crossed an ocean with ambition and almost no financial literacy. I am a nurse who worked two jobs and only realized too late what overtime was actually costing. And I am also — because I chose it, because I did the work, because I refused to let the inherited story be the final one — a healthcare executive, an entrepreneur, a PhD candidate, a business owner operating across two continents, a mother who picks her children up from school, a woman whose overtime is a choice.

Both of those people are real. The first one is where I started. The second one is what I built. And the bridge between them was not a single dramatic moment of transformation. It was the daily, unglamorous decision to stop performing a financial identity and start building a real one.

What the Real Story Sounds Like

Not: 'I am fine. I just like to keep busy.'

But: 'I am building something. I am not there yet. I am on my way.'

Not: 'I picked up the overtime because I wanted to.'

But: 'I am working toward the day when overtime is optional — and I have a plan.'

Not: 'Money has never been my thing.'

But: 'Money was never taught to me. I am teaching it to myself now.'

The real story is not weaker than the performance. It is braver.

The Cultural Weight of Sending Money Home

I want to acknowledge something that sits at the intersection of identity, culture, and financial reality for a significant portion of the nurses reading this book: the obligation — financial, emotional, and deeply cultural — of supporting family in another country.

For immigrant nurses, this is not an optional line item in the budget. It is a responsibility understood before you left, part of the implicit contract of the opportunity you were given, and one that carries a weight no spreadsheet fully captures. The school fees. The medical expenses. The sibling who needs support while they complete their education. The parent whose retirement did not look like the one they deserved. These are real obligations, carried by real people, across real distances, often in silence because the complexity of holding them while also trying to build your own financial life is too nuanced to explain to someone who has not lived it.

I have lived it. And I want to say this plainly: the fact that you carry this does not make you less capable of building wealth. It makes the building harder and the intentionality more non-negotiable. You are not managing one financial life. You are managing the downstream effects of your success on multiple people who are counting on you. That is not a burden to be ashamed of. It is a responsibility to be managed with the same strategic clarity you bring to everything else in this book.

Name the obligation. Put it in the budget. Give it its honest number. And then build the income and the assets that make it sustainable — not because you resent it, but because the people depending on you deserve the version of you that has her own financial life intact, not the version who is quietly drowning while sending money home.

> ***You cannot pour from an empty account any more than from an empty cup. Building your own financial foundation is not selfishness. It is sustainability.***

Taking the Mask Off — What Healing Actually Looks Like

Healing your financial identity does not happen in a seminar or on a single Saturday when you reorganize your accounts. It happens in the small, repeated moments when you choose honesty over performance — when you tell the truth to yourself before you worry about what it looks like to anyone else.

It looks like this: you look at next month's schedule and see that you have agreed to three overtime shifts out of habit and exhaustion management, rather than by intention. And instead of telling yourself the familiar story — I want to, I like the extra hours — you say the real one: I agreed to these because I felt financial pressure. I am going to use this income intentionally rather than let it disappear, as it usually does.

It looks like this: a colleague mentions she is starting to invest, and instead of deflecting with the usual vague response, you say, "I have been learning about that too," and ask her what she has found useful. One honest sentence opens a conversation that the performance would have closed. That conversation may be the one that changes your trajectory.

It looks like this: you sit down with the net worth worksheet from Chapter 2, and you look at it without shame — not as a verdict on who you are, but as a precise description of where you are starting from. You have been further from a goal before. You have closed harder gaps. You know how to work toward something difficult. This is not different. This is just financial.

The Daily Practice of Financial Honesty

Once a week, look at your actual spending from the past seven days — without judgment, with accuracy.

Once a month, update your net worth calculation and note the direction of change.

When overtime is offered, ask honestly: do I want this or do I need this? Answer yourself truthfully.

When you catch yourself performing financial wellness — in conversation, on social media, internally — pause and ask what the true sentence would be.

Find one person in your life — one — with whom you can be financially honest. Not to expose yourself. To stop being alone with it.

Financial healing is not a solo act. But it begins with a solo decision: to stop lying to yourself.

The Nurse Who Tells the Truth

I want to close this chapter by describing the version of you that is possible on the other side of this work. Not a perfect version. Not a version without financial complexity or cultural obligation or the occasional hard month. But a version that has made a different kind of decision about her relationship with money and with the stories she tells about it.

She does not pretend the overtime is a choice when it is not — because she has done the work to make it an actual choice, and the distance between those two realities is now too meaningful to collapse with a casual performance. When she picks up an extra shift, it is because she has a specific reason — a goal named, a destination assigned — and she can say so without embarrassment.

She carries her cultural obligations with love rather than resentment, because she has built a financial structure that accounts for them rather than absorbing them in silence. She is not prioritizing her family's financial well-being back home. She is actually building it.

She talks about money differently than she used to — not with shame, and not with the exhausting performance of having figured it all out, but with the quiet confidence of someone who is engaged with her financial life rather than hiding from it. She has opinions. She has a plan. She has made mistakes, learned from them, and is not defined by them.

She is further along than she was. She knows where she is going. And she got there not by waiting until she had enough or knew enough or had the perfect moment — but by taking the mask off, looking honestly at what was actually there, and deciding to build something real.

> ***The most powerful financial decision you will ever make is the one you make in private — when you stop performing and start being honest about exactly where you are and exactly where you intend to go.***

This Is Where the Healing Begins

Every chapter in this book has given you a tool. A budget framework. A debt elimination strategy. An investment principle. A way to think about overtime, time, presence, and legacy.

This chapter gives you something different. It gives you permission — permission to stop maintaining a financial performance that is costing you the energy you need to build a real financial life. Permission to tell the truth about where you are without shame. Permission to be in the middle of the journey and say so. Permission to need help and seek it. Permission to have started in a different place than the people around you and to be building toward a different destination without pretending the starting point was the same.

You are not behind. You are not broken. You are not the sum of the financial mistakes you have made, the season you are in, or the gap that still exists between where you are and where you want to be. You are a person in motion — a clinician, a builder, a woman who crossed oceans, held families together, showed up for patients, and kept going on days when keeping going was all that was available.

You are also, as of this chapter, someone who has decided to stop lying about the cost of all that keeping going. Someone who has looked at overtime not as a badge of honor but as a symptom with a treatable cause. Someone who has chosen honesty over performance because she finally understands that the performance was never protecting her. It was just keeping her stuck.

The mask is heavy. You have been carrying it for a long time.

Set it down.

Build something real instead.

To Every Nurse Who Has Ever Said 'I'm Fine' When She Wasn't

You were not weak for carrying it.

You were not wrong for protecting the image while you figured things out.

But you no longer have to carry it.

The truth — your actual financial truth, wherever it stands today — is not your enemy.

It is the only foundation strong enough to build on.

Start there. Start now. Start honest.

Heal Your Wealth — Chapter 9 Reflection

This is the most personal chapter in this book. These questions are not designed to be comfortable. They are designed to be true. Answer them in writing, privately, with the same courage it took to pick up this book in the first place.

1. In the past month, how many times did you frame overtime or extra work as a choice when it was driven by financial necessity? Write down the honest version of one of those moments. Not to judge it — to see it clearly.
2. What is the financial reality you have never said out loud to anyone? Write it here, in this private space, in one plain sentence. The balance, the debt, the gap, the fear — whatever it is. Say it to yourself first.
3. What is the money story you inherited — from your family, your culture, your upbringing? Write it down as a sentence your parents or guardians lived by, even if they never said it explicitly. Then ask: Is this still my story? Does it still serve me?
4. Is there one person in your life with whom you could have a genuine, unperformed conversation about money? Not to expose your full balance sheet — but to stop being completely alone with the reality. Who is that person? What would you say if you were being honest?
5. Write the financial identity statement you are choosing going forward — not the inherited one, not the performed one, but the one you are actively building. Start it with: 'I am a person who...' and complete it with something true, specific, and forward-facing.

The mask is heavy. You have been carrying it for a long time. This is the chapter where you set it down — not in front of anyone else, but in front of yourself. That is where all real healing begins.

— — —

In Chapter 10, we protect what you are building because wealth without protection is a sandcastle — beautiful, temporary, and entirely vulnerable to the first storm. Disability insurance, liability coverage, estate planning, and the legal and financial instruments that ensure that what you have worked for survives the unexpected. The chapter most people skip because it feels premature. The chapter that matters most when something goes wrong.

You have taken the mask off. Now, let us make sure what is underneath it is built to last.

Continue to Chapter 10: Protecting Your Wealth

CHAPTER TEN

Protecting Your Wealth

Your degree is a lifetime legacy. So is everything you build with it. Protect both.

Imagine a nurse who spent fifteen years building her financial life with extraordinary discipline.

She paid off her student loans. She eliminated her credit card debt. She bought a home in a good neighborhood and steadily built equity. She maxed her 403(b) every year for a decade, opened a Roth IRA, and started a small rental property portfolio that generated income every month without requiring additional shifts. She earned her NP credential and significantly increased her income. She invested in certifications, attended conferences, and built a clinical reputation that opened executive doors. She did, in other words, almost everything this book has described.

And then she sustained a back injury that ended her clinical practice for fourteen months.

She had no disability insurance. She had no income replacement. The rental properties helped—but not enough to cover the mortgage, family obligations, living expenses, and the mounting medical costs simultaneously. She withdrew from her retirement account early, triggering penalties and taxes that cost her tens of thousands of dollars she had built over the years. The emergency fund, carefully maintained, lasted four months. By month six, she was in territory that looked uncomfortably like the paycheck-to-paycheck life she had spent fifteen years escaping.

The building was real. The protection was absent. And the absence of protection undid, in months, what had taken years to construct.

> ***You can build extraordinary wealth and lose it to a single unprotected event. Protection is not a luxury you add after you have enough. It is the structure that makes the building permanent.***

Your Degree Is a Lifetime Asset — Insure It Accordingly

Before we discuss protecting the money, we need to talk about protecting the mechanism that generates it: your clinical credential and your ability to practice.

Your nursing degree, your NP licensure, your specialty certifications, your clinical reputation — these are assets. They are the assets that produce all the other assets described in this book. Without the ability to practice, the income stops. Without the income, the investments stop growing, the mortgage payments stop arriving, and the family obligations become impossible to meet. The most valuable thing you own is not your property or your retirement account. It is your capacity to generate income using the skills you spent years acquiring.

Protecting that capacity requires attention on two fronts: maintaining the credential itself and ensuring it can be used.

License Protection — The Basics You Cannot Afford to Neglect

Your clinical license is the gate through which all earnings pass. Losing it — through a disciplinary action, a lapse in renewal, or a scope-of-practice violation — is the most financially catastrophic event that most healthcare professionals never plan for. And yet the majority of clinicians have no specific plan for license defense, no legal protection policy, and no understanding of how quickly a complaint — even an unfounded one — can drain personal resources through legal fees alone.

Protecting Your Clinical License — Non-Negotiable Steps

Renew on time, every time: Set calendar reminders twelve weeks before expiration — never allow a lapse.

Maintain continuing education requirements: Track CE credits throughout the cycle, not in the final month.

Document everything: Patient encounters, decisions, communications — the chart is your legal protection.

Understand your scope of practice in every state you practice: Especially critical for multi-state NPs and telehealth providers.

Carry professional liability (malpractice) insurance: Even if your employer provides coverage, a personal policy protects you in the event your employer's coverage is unavailable.

Consider a license defense rider or legal protection policy: NSO (Nurses Service Organization) and similar providers offer affordable coverage.

Report disciplinary issues immediately and consult an attorney: Early legal counsel is exponentially less expensive than late legal counsel.

Your license is your most valuable professional asset. Treat its protection with the same attention you give your investments.

Disability Insurance: The Coverage Most Healthcare Workers Are Missing

Disability insurance is the most important insurance product that most healthcare professionals do not have—or have in amounts so inadequate that it would not actually protect them if the need arose.

The statistics are sobering. According to the Social Security Administration, more than one in four workers will experience a disability that prevents them from working for ninety days or more before they reach retirement age. For healthcare workers — who are among the most physically demanding workforces in any economy — the risk is not theoretical. Back injuries, repetitive stress conditions, needlestick exposures, the cumulative physical toll of years of long shifts: these are real risks, lived by real clinicians, that end or interrupt careers with a regularity the profession rarely discusses openly.

The question is not whether disability could happen. The question is whether you have built the financial infrastructure to survive it without dismantling everything you have built.

Understanding What Your Employer's Coverage Actually Provides

Many healthcare employers offer short- and long-term disability coverage as part of their benefits package. Before you assume you are covered, read the policy carefully — because the coverage your employer provides and the coverage you actually need may be significantly different.

Real-Life Scenario: The Gap in Employer Coverage

Sarah is an NP earning $115,000 per year at a nonprofit hospital.

Her employer provides long-term disability coverage at 60% of salary after a 90-day elimination period.

60% of $115,000 = $69,000 per year, or $5,750 per month before taxes.

Her monthly essential expenses: mortgage $2,200, car $450, utilities $300, childcare $1,400, family remittance $600, food $600 = $5,550 per month minimum.

Result: Sarah's employer coverage barely covers her floor — with nothing for medical costs, debt payments, retirement contributions, or any buffer.

A supplemental individual disability policy would bridge that gap.

Lesson: Employer coverage is the starting point. It is rarely the complete answer.

What to Look for in a Disability Insurance Policy

When evaluating disability insurance — whether reviewing an employer policy or shopping for an individual one — these are the variables that determine whether the coverage will actually protect you.

Policy Feature	What It Means	What to Look For
Elimination period	How long before benefits begin	90 days is standard; shorter costs more but protects earlier
Benefit period	How long benefits are paid	To age 65 or lifetime — not a fixed 2 or 5 years
Benefit amount	Monthly income replacement	60–80% of gross income; supplement employer coverage to reach this
Own-occupation definition	Pays if you cannot do YOUR specific job	Critical for NPs and specialists — not just 'any occupation'
Non-cancelable / guaranteed renewable	Insurer cannot change terms	Essential for long-term protection
COLA rider	Benefit increases with inflation	Important for policies held 10+ years
Future increase option	Add coverage as income grows without re-exam	Valuable for clinicians early in career growth
Partial / residual disability	Pays if partially disabled	Protects if you can work reduced hours only

The own-occupation definition deserves particular emphasis for advanced practice providers. A policy with an 'any occupation' definition pays only if you cannot perform any job at all — meaning a nurse practitioner who cannot perform clinical duties but could theoretically answer phones would not qualify. A true own-occupation policy pays if you cannot perform the specific duties of your clinical role, regardless of whether you could do something else. For a clinician whose specialized training represents years of investment, nothing less than own-occupation coverage is adequate.

Life Insurance: Protecting the People Who Depend on You

If anyone in your life depends on your income — children, a spouse or partner, aging parents, family members whose support relies on your earnings — life insurance is not optional. It is the mechanism by which the financial life you have built continues to function for the people it was built for, even if you are not there to sustain it.

The question most people get wrong about life insurance is not whether they need it but how much they need. The standard rule of thumb — ten to twelve times your annual income — is a reasonable starting point. Still, it requires adjustment for the specific obligations of the healthcare professional: student loan balances that might be passed to cosigners, family remittances that would end abruptly, mortgage balances on properties you own, and the support of children through education and early adulthood.

Term vs. Whole Life: The Decision Healthcare Professionals Get Sold Wrong

The insurance industry generates significant commission income from whole life insurance, which is why it is aggressively sold to professionals who a different approach would better serve. Let me be direct about what most financial advisors who receive insurance commissions do not tell you: for most healthcare professionals, especially those in the building phase of their financial lives, term life insurance is the appropriate product.

Term vs. Whole Life — The Plain Truth

TERM LIFE INSURANCE:

Pure death benefit for a defined period (10, 20, or 30 years)

Premiums are significantly lower for equivalent coverage amounts

Best for: protecting income and obligations during the years they exist

A healthy NP in her 30s can secure $1,000,000 of term coverage for $40–60/month

WHOLE LIFE INSURANCE:

Permanent coverage with a cash value component

Premiums are 5–15x higher than equivalent term coverage

Cash value growth is typically slower than a low-cost index fund

Best for: specific estate planning situations, usually for high-net-worth individuals

Often sold as an 'investment' — it is not a substitute for actual investments

The right answer for most clinicians: Buy term. Invest the difference.

A $50/month whole life premium can buy $1M of term — and $400/month into a Roth IRA.

Twenty years later, the Roth significantly outperforms the whole life cash value.

Professional Liability: Your Clinical Shield

Every healthcare professional who provides direct patient care is exposed to malpractice liability. A single lawsuit — even one that is ultimately dismissed — can cost tens of thousands of dollars in legal fees, consume years of professional and emotional energy, and in severe cases result in judgments that threaten personal assets if coverage is inadequate.

Many clinicians rely entirely on their employer's malpractice coverage. This is a significant vulnerability, for a simple reason: your employer's policy covers you while you are acting on their behalf. If you do any clinical work outside that employment —

independent consulting, volunteer healthcare work, moonlighting, telehealth through a separate platform — you may have no coverage at all for claims arising from those activities. And if your employment ends, your coverage ends with it for events that occurred during that employment, unless you carry a tail policy.

Real-Life Scenario: The Gap in Employer Malpractice Coverage

Marcus is a PA employed full-time at a multi-specialty clinic.
He also provides weekend telehealth consultations through a separate platform.
His employer's malpractice coverage applies only to the clinic employment.
A patient files a complaint arising from a telehealth encounter.
Marcus has no coverage for this claim. Legal defense alone costs $45,000.
The matter is eventually resolved, but the financial and emotional toll is significant.

Lesson: Every clinical activity needs coverage. Not just the primary employment.
An individual professional liability policy from NSO or HPSO costs approximately $100–300/year for most advanced practice providers. It is not optional.

Occurrence vs. Claims-Made: The Distinction That Matters

When evaluating malpractice insurance, the policy type determines what happens when you change jobs or retire. An occurrence policy covers any event that occurs during the policy period, regardless of when the claim is filed, even years later. A claims-made policy covers only claims filed while the policy is active. If you leave an employer with claims-made coverage and do not purchase a tail policy, you have no coverage for claims filed after your departure, even if the incident occurred while you were there. This gap has ended careers and depleted savings for healthcare professionals who did not understand the distinction until a claim arrived.

Estate Planning: The Documents That Protect Everything

Estate planning is the category of wealth protection that healthcare professionals most consistently defer to — and the one whose absence causes the most preventable damage to families when something goes wrong. The clinician who has spent a career building wealth, only to leave it unprotected by basic legal documents, has inadvertently created a situation where the state, rather than her intentions, determines what happens to everything she built.

Estate planning is not exclusively for the elderly or the extraordinarily wealthy. It is for anyone who has assets, dependents, or specific wishes about what should happen to both. If you own property, have children, have retirement accounts, have a business interest, or have family members in another country who depend on your support, you need estate planning documents. Not eventually. Now.

The Core Estate Planning Documents Every Healthcare Professional Needs

1. WILL (Last Will and Testament)

Directs the distribution of your assets upon death.

Names a guardian for minor children — without this, a court decides.

Without a will, your state's intestacy laws determine who gets what, which may not align with your wishes or your family's needs.

2. DURABLE POWER OF ATTORNEY (Financial)

Designates someone to manage your financial affairs if you are incapacitated.

Without this, a court must appoint a conservator—a costly and time-consuming process.

Critical for clinicians who could be injured or ill for an extended period.

3. HEALTHCARE POWER OF ATTORNEY / HEALTHCARE PROXY

Names someone to make medical decisions if you cannot make them yourself.

Every clinician who has seen families in conflict over an incapacitated patient understands why this document exists. Do not leave your family without it.

4. ADVANCE DIRECTIVE / LIVING WILL

Specifies your wishes for end-of-life care.

As a clinician, you know what these decisions look like from the other side.

Document your wishes so no one has to guess.

5. BENEFICIARY DESIGNATIONS (not a document, but equally critical)

Retirement accounts, life insurance, and some bank accounts pass by beneficiary designation — outside of your will entirely.

Review and update after every major life change: marriage, divorce, birth, death.

A misnamed beneficiary can override an entire will.

The Trust: When It Makes Sense for Healthcare Professionals

A revocable living trust is an estate planning tool that allows assets to pass to your beneficiaries without going through probate — the court-supervised process that validates a will and distributes an estate. Probate is public, slow, and costly. A trust bypasses it entirely, meaning your estate can be distributed according to your wishes promptly and privately.

For healthcare professionals who own real estate in multiple states, operate a business, or have international beneficiaries — family members in Kenya, Nigeria, the Philippines, or anywhere outside the United States — a trust is particularly valuable. Multi-state property passing through probate must be handled separately in each state. A trust avoids this entirely.

Real-Life Scenario: The Will That Was Not Enough

Dr. Amara, an ER physician, owned a primary home in Texas, a rental property in Georgia, and a small business interest. She had a will but no trust.

When she died unexpectedly at 51, her estate had to go through probate in both Texas and Georgia.

The dual-state probate process took 22 months and cost her estate over $40,000 in legal fees.

Her business interests were frozen during the process, resulting in lost revenue that her family depended on.

Her international beneficiaries — her parents in Nigeria — faced additional complications transferring funds across borders without the trust structure that would have simplified it.

Lesson: A will directs how assets are distributed. A trust controls how they get there.

For clinicians with property in multiple states or international beneficiaries, a revocable living trust is worth every dollar of the legal fee to establish it.

Asset Protection: Shielding What You Have Built

Asset protection is the legal strategy of structuring your financial life so that a lawsuit, a creditor claim, or a business liability cannot reach your personal wealth. For healthcare professionals — who operate in one of the highest-liability professional environments that exists — this is not paranoia. It is prudence.

Healthcare professionals are among the most sued professionals in any economy. Malpractice claims, employment disputes, business disagreements, and personal liability from investment properties all represent potential pathways through which your personal assets can be threatened. The goal of asset protection is not to hide wealth or evade legitimate obligations. It is to ensure that a professional liability does not become a personal financial catastrophe.

The LLC for Investment Properties

If you own rental properties, holding them inside a Limited Liability Company is one of the most straightforward and widely used asset protection strategies available to individual investors. An LLC creates a legal separation between the property and your personal assets — meaning that if a tenant sues over a slip-and-fall on your rental property, the lawsuit can reach the LLC's assets but generally cannot reach your personal bank account, your primary home, or your retirement savings.

Each property, or each geographic cluster of properties, should ideally be held in a separate LLC to prevent a claim against one property from threatening the equity in another. The cost to establish and maintain an LLC varies by state. Still, it is typically a few hundred dollars annually — an extraordinarily inexpensive form of insurance against multi-million-dollar personal liability exposure.

The Business Entity for Clinical Entrepreneurship

If you run a clinical practice, a consulting business, a staffing company, or any other healthcare business as a sole proprietor — meaning under your own name without a separate legal entity — your personal assets are exposed to every business liability that arises. A disgruntled client, a contract dispute, an employment claim from a staff member: any of these could reach your personal savings, your home, your investment accounts.

Operating through an LLC, a Professional LLC (PLLC), an S-Corporation, or another appropriate business structure separates your personal wealth from your business liability. It also, depending on the structure, creates tax efficiency that reduces the percentage of business income going to the government — a secondary benefit that compounds meaningfully over a career of entrepreneurship.

Real-Life Scenario: The Consultant Who Had No Entity

Priya, an NP with deep expertise in quality improvement, began consulting for hospital systems

on the side of her primary employment. She billed under her own name as a sole proprietor.

One hospital client disputed a deliverable and filed a breach-of-contract claim for $85,000.

Because Priya had no business entity, the claim was against her personally.

Her personal savings, her car, and her investment accounts were all potentially reachable.

She settled for $30,000 — money that came from the savings account she had built with discipline.

A PLLC or LLC, established before the consulting work began,

would have limited the claim to the business entity's assets — not her personal wealth.

The entity setup cost: approximately $300-500 in most states.

The cost of not having it: $30,000 and significant stress.

Umbrella Insurance: The Most Underused Protection Tool

A personal umbrella insurance policy provides liability coverage above and beyond the limits of your home, auto, and other policies. For a premium of approximately $200 to $400 per year, a one to two million dollar umbrella policy covers you against major liability claims that could otherwise penetrate your personal assets — a serious car accident, a guest injured on your property, a lawsuit arising from personal activity rather than professional practice.

For healthcare professionals with growing net worth, an umbrella policy is one of the highest-value protection tools available per dollar of premium. The coverage amount should increase as your net worth increases — a rule of thumb is to carry umbrella coverage at least equal to your total net worth.

Retirement Planning: The Long View of Protection

Every chapter of this book has been about building. This section is about ensuring that what you build is accessible — on your terms, at the time you choose — when you arrive at the season for which all of it was constructed.

Retirement planning for healthcare professionals requires a longer horizon than most planning tools assume, because healthcare professionals often enter their peak earning years later than other professionals — the years of training, credentialing, and student loan management delay compounding that begins earlier for other professionals. A nurse practitioner who graduated at 30 and spent years paying down debt before beginning serious investing may be 40 before the wealth-building phase truly accelerates. The retirement timeline compresses, making every decision in the intervening years more consequential.

The Retirement Protection Checklist

What Retirement Security Actually Requires — Beyond the 403(b)

INCOME REPLACEMENT (aim for 80% of pre-retirement income):

Employer retirement account (403b/401k) maximized — the foundation
Roth IRA contributing consistently — the tax-free growth layer
Taxable investment account for pre-retirement access — the bridge
Rental income — passive income that does not require liquidating investments
Social Security — understand your projected benefit; do not rely on it exclusively

HEALTHCARE COVERAGE (the retirement risk most people do not plan for):

Medicare begins at 65 — if you retire before 65, private coverage is required
Medicare supplement (Medigap) policy for costs Medicare does not cover
Long-term care insurance — nursing home costs average $90,000+ per year
Health Savings Account (HSA) — triple tax advantage; invest for retirement healthcare

LIFESTYLE PROTECTION:

Emergency fund maintained in retirement — 12 months of expenses minimum
Home paid off or equity plan in place before retirement
Estate plan updated — beneficiaries reviewed, will and trust current
Annual review with a fee-only financial advisor

INCOME SEQUENCING (which accounts for drawing from and when):

Draw taxable accounts first (no penalty, manage capital gains)
Then tax-deferred accounts (traditional 403b/401k — taxed as income)
Roth IRA last — it grows tax-free and has no required minimum distributions
Rental income runs in parallel throughout — reduces pressure on investment accounts

The vision of retirement for the healthcare professional who has built intentionally is not a sudden stop—a cliff where the work ends and a quiet emptiness begins. It is a transition. Clinical practice becomes consulting. The investment portfolio generates income. The rental properties produce cash flow. The business you built creates ongoing revenue that does not require your daily presence. The retirement you arrive at is not the end of earning. It is the beginning of earning on your own terms, funded by the decisions you made in every chapter that led to this one.

> ***The life you built is waiting for you on the other side of the career. The only question is whether you protected it well enough to receive it intact.***

The Annual Wealth Protection Review

Wealth protection is not a one-time event. It is an annual practice — the equivalent of a physical examination for your financial life. Things change: income grows, properties are acquired, families expand, laws shift, and the coverage that was adequate three years ago may be dangerously insufficient today.

Every year, sit down with your financial picture and run through the complete protection review. Not with anxiety — with the same clinical precision you bring to a patient's annual assessment. Identify what has changed. Update what needs updating. Close any gaps that have opened. And document the review, so that next year you are not starting from zero.

The Annual Wealth Protection Review — Your Checklist

INSURANCE REVIEW:

Is my disability coverage still adequate for my current income?

Is my life insurance sufficient for my current obligations?

Are my malpractice and license defense policies current and appropriately scoped?

Do I have umbrella coverage? Is the limit still equal to or greater than my net worth?

Have I reviewed my homeowner's and landlord policies this year?

ESTATE PLAN REVIEW:

Has my will been updated in the past 3–5 years?

Are all beneficiary designations current — especially after any life change?

If I have a trust, are all the intended assets properly titled in the trust name?

Do my healthcare proxy and power of attorney documents reflect my current wishes?

LEGAL STRUCTURE REVIEW:
Are my investment properties held in appropriate legal entities?
Is my consulting or business income flowing through a proper business structure?
Have I consulted a tax professional about the most efficient entity structure for my income level?

RETIREMENT TRAJECTORY REVIEW:
Am I on track for the retirement income I need? Run the projection.
Have I maxed all available tax-advantaged contributions this year?
Is my investment allocation still appropriate for my timeline?

Schedule this review at the same time every year. Put it in your calendar now.

The Day You Retire — What It Should Look Like

I want you to hold a vision. Not an abstract one — a specific, detailed, fully imagined vision of what the day you step back from clinical practice should feel like, if you have protected everything you built with the diligence this chapter describes.

You wake up that morning without an alarm. The mortgage is paid, or the rental income covers it. The children you raised in the neighborhood you chose deliberately are launched — educated, stable, carrying the model of ownership and intentionality you modeled for them through every financial decision you made. The retirement accounts you began building in your thirties have compounded for three decades and now generate income that arrives monthly without requiring your clinical hours to sustain it. The properties you acquired — the primary home, the investment units, perhaps the commercial space that houses a business — are assets that belong to your family and will continue to belong to them after you are gone.

You have a will that reflects your current wishes. You have a trust that will spare your family the cost and delay of probate. You have life insurance that would have protected your dependents if anything had happened along the way — and didn't need to be claimed, which is the best possible outcome. You have a financial advisor who knows your complete picture and has helped you sequence your accounts so that taxes in retirement are as low as legally achievable.

You have access to the life you built. Not a diminished version of it. Not a scramble to cover gaps that proper planning would have prevented. The full thing — intact, funded, protected, and passed forward to the generation that is watching what you built and learning, as children always do, from the model rather than the instruction.

That day is not guaranteed. But it is buildable. It has been buildable from the very first chapter of this book. And the protection this chapter describes is the final layer—the seal that makes it durable.

What You Are Protecting When You Protect Your Wealth

The fifteen years of discipline that eliminated the debt.
The down payment saved from the income of intentional shifts.
The equity built in the home where your children grew up.
The retirement account that compounded quietly while you were focused on living.
The business you built from clinical expertise and the refusal to settle.
The family in Kenya whose school fees you paid across an ocean, with love.
The generation that is watching you — and will build their own version of this because they saw you build yours.

Heal Your Wealth — Chapter 10 Reflection

Building wealth without protecting it is like earning a clinical credential and never renewing your license. The work you did to get here deserves the structure that keeps it safe. Answer these questions with that seriousness.

6. Do you currently carry individual disability insurance with an own-occupation definition? If not, research three providers this month — Principal, Guardian, and MassMutual are among the most reputable for healthcare professionals — and get a quote. Know the premium before you decide not to have it.
7. Pull out every insurance policy you currently hold: life, disability, malpractice, homeowners, and auto. For each one, write down the coverage amount and ask whether that amount still reflects your current net worth and obligations. Identify the gap.
8. Do you have a will? Have you reviewed it in the past three years? Have your beneficiary designations been updated after every major life change — marriage, children, divorce, death of a named beneficiary? Address every no answer before moving to the next chapter.
9. If you own investment properties or operate any consulting or clinical business outside your primary employment, are those activities held inside a proper legal entity? If not, consult a business attorney or legal services platform this month. The cost of the entity is a fraction of the cost of the liability it prevents.
10. Write the retirement vision in full — not as a financial projection, but as a day. What does the morning look like when you no longer need to work? Where are you? Who is with you? What does the financial infrastructure that makes that morning possible look like? Write it in enough detail that it becomes a destination rather than an abstraction.

Your degree is a lifetime legacy. So is every investment, every property, every dollar you have built with discipline and intention. Protect all of it — with the same rigor you brought to earning it.

— — —

In the final chapter, we lift our eyes from the mechanics of building and protecting and turn toward what all of it is ultimately for: the legacy. The financial story that outlasts your career, that your children carry forward, that the profession is shaped by because you were in it and refused to accept that financial struggle was a permanent condition of clinical work.

You have built something. You have protected it. Now let us talk about what you leave behind—and how to make sure it carries the full weight of everything you poured into it.

Continue to Chapter 11: Your Financial Legacy

CHAPTER ELEVEN

Your Financial Legacy

What you build today becomes the foundation someone else stands on tomorrow

There is a question I want to ask you before we begin this final chapter — not as a rhetorical device, but as a genuine inquiry that I hope you will sit with before you read another word.

What do you want your financial life to say about you when you are no longer building it?

Not the balance in the account. Not the properties on the deed or the certificates on the wall. But the story — the one your children absorb before they are old enough to articulate it, the one your community reads in how you show up, the one your profession inherits because you were in it and chose to do something different with what you earned. What do you want that story to say?

I have thought about this question for years — while I was deep in the overtime trap and could not yet see the way out, while I was studying for board exams at midnight after a full clinical day, while I was building Icon Oncology Supply and learning what it means to build something that serves people in two countries simultaneously, while I was raising children who were watching everything I did with the attention that children give to the adults who shape their understanding of what is possible.

Here is what I want my financial life to say: that I did what I loved, without having to work beyond my capacity to sustain it. That my children grew up knowing how to build and sustain wealth — not because I lectured them about it, but because they watched me live it. That I gave them the opportunity I was never afforded: financial knowledge, a model, a head start. And that is when I look back at the life I built – from a childhood in Kenya through an IT career, through nursing school, through an executive suite, and across two continents—I would not change the work. I would have started the financial literacy sooner.

> ***Legacy is not what you accumulate. Legacy is what you transfer — the wealth, the wisdom, and the model of what is possible for people who come from where you came from.***

The Freedom to Do What You Love

The financial legacy I am building is not primarily about a number. It is about a condition: the freedom to spend my professional energy on meaningful work, without financial pressure forcing me into merely available work.

That distinction — meaningful versus merely available — is one of the most important in this entire book. Every nurse who has taken a shift she did not want because she needed the income understands it. Every clinician who has stayed in a role that no longer served her growth because the salary was too reliable to leave understands it. Every healthcare professional who has had an idea for a business, a book, a clinical program, a global health initiative — and has not pursued it because the financial margin for risk was too thin — understands it.

Financial freedom does not mean you stop working. It means you stop being forced to work in ways that diminish you. It means the clinical work you choose to do matters, uses your gifts at their highest level, and connects you to the patients, the problems, and the purpose that called you into healthcare in the first place. Not because the mortgage autopays on Monday and the account needs to be there.

That freedom is the goal. Not the retirement account balance. Not the net worth figure. The freedom. The choosing. Showing up to work because you want to — and knowing, on the days when you do not want to, that you could step back and the financial infrastructure would hold.

MY FINANCIAL LEGACY STATEMENT

To do what I love, without being forced by financial necessity.

To give my children what I was never given: the knowledge, the model, and the head start.

To prove, by the way I lived, that APRNs can build generational wealth.

To leave the profession better than I found it — and the family further than I started.

Raising Children Who Know How to Build

My children will not struggle with financial literacy the way I did. Not because I will shelter them from the reality of money, but because I will teach them to face it directly, with knowledge and without shame, from the earliest age at which the conversation makes sense.

That teaching is not primarily a curriculum. It is a model. Children do not learn their deepest financial beliefs from conversations. They learn them from observation — from watching what the adults in their lives do with money, from absorbing the emotional temperature of financial decisions, and from understanding, through daily life, whether money is a source of anxiety or a tool managed with intention and confidence.

When my children see me review my investment accounts, they learn that investing is normal. When they watch me make a deliberate decision about a purchase — not impulsively, not with guilt, but with the clear assessment of whether it aligns with the plan — they learn that spending can be intentional rather than reflexive. When they see that I work because I find the work meaningful, not because I am desperate for the income it produces, they absorb a model of professional life that is entirely different from the one I grew up watching.

That model — lived rather than taught — is the most durable financial inheritance I can give them. More durable than any account, any property, any dollar amount. Because the knowledge of how to build transfers forward in ways that assets alone do not. An inheritance of money without the knowledge of how to manage and grow it is spent within a generation. An inheritance of financial wisdom compounds indefinitely.

What I Am Teaching My Children About Money

That wealth is built — not inherited, not lucky, not reserved for other people.

That debt is a tool when used strategically, and a trap when used unconsciously.

That the overtime trap is real, and the way out is intentionality — not more hours.

That a credential is a platform, not a destination.

That real estate, invested well, generates income while you sleep.

That your financial story is not fixed by where you started.

That people from Kenya can build companies that operate in multiple countries.

That APRNs can do this, too — all of it.

The Opportunity I Was Never Afforded — That I Am Giving Forward

I grew up in a household where money was managed, not mastered. Where the paycheck arrived, the obligations consumed it, and what remained was small, unreliable, and never enough to build anything permanent. Not because my parents were irresponsible. Because they had never been taught anything different. The knowledge was absent. The model was survival. And survival, normalized across enough generations, stops feeling like a temporary condition and starts feeling like the permanent state of people like us.

I refuse that inheritance. I refused it when I paid off my debt. I refused it when I bought my home in a neighborhood I chose for my children, rather than one that was convenient for my budget. I refused it when I built a company that operates across East Africa. I refuse it every time I sit down with this book and put into words the financial knowledge that no one handed me — so that someone else might not have to find it the long way, the way I did.

The opportunity I was never afforded was simple: someone who looked like me, who had come from where I came from, sitting down and saying, "Here is how this works." Here is the credit card trap. Here is the overtime revolving door. Here is what the employer match actually means and why you are leaving money on the table. Here is what your credentials can do beyond the first job. Here is how to buy a home, protect it, and build above it. Here is how to raise children who do not start from zero, the way you did.

This book is that conversation. The one I wish I had been given. Offered now to every nurse, every NP, every PA, every pharmacist, every therapist, every allied health professional who is brilliant and hardworking and underserved by the financial education system — and who deserves better than the overtime trap as a permanent condition of clinical excellence.

> ***I could not be given this knowledge at the beginning. So I built it across a career and wrote it down so that someone starting today does not have to wait as long as I did to find it.***

The Entrepreneurial Legacy — Building Something That Outlasts You

Legacy, for the entrepreneur clinician, is more expansive than a retirement account and a paid-off mortgage. It is the business that continues to generate value after you have stepped back from the daily operations. The platform that serves patients, professionals, or communities in ways that were not possible before you built it. The team you developed, whose careers were shaped by the leadership you modeled. The intellectual property — the book, the course, the clinical protocol, the research contribution — that becomes part of the professional landscape in ways that persist long after the author has moved on.

Icon Oncology Supply is part of my entrepreneurial legacy. A company that began with a vision of improving access to oncology and dialysis medications in underserved markets now operates across East Africa and serves patients who would otherwise go without the treatments that, in clinical training, I have been taught are the difference between suffering and dignity. That company will outlast my daily involvement in it. The patients it serves, the infrastructure it builds, the pharmaceutical access it creates in chronically underserved markets — that is a legacy that a paycheck never produces.

Every healthcare professional with an entrepreneurial vision can build something with this kind of reach. The clinical credential is the credibility. Knowledge of the system's gaps is market research. The discipline built through years of managing complex clinical environments is operational competence. What is needed is the courage to begin—and the financial foundation that makes it possible without catastrophic personal risk.

The Entrepreneur Clinician's Legacy Blueprint

WHAT TO BUILD:

A business that solves a problem you identified from inside the healthcare system

A platform that generates income independently of your daily hours

An intellectual property asset — book, course, protocol — that carries your knowledge forward

A team that grows under your leadership and carries the mission beyond your personal capacity

HOW TO FUND IT (the financially responsible sequence):

Step 1: Personal debt eliminated — you cannot build for others while sinking personally

Step 2: Emergency fund in place — 6 months of personal expenses before business risk

Step 3: Start the business as a side endeavor while the primary income is stable

Step 4: Reinvest early profits into the business — not into personal lifestyle expansion

Step 5: Scale deliberately, with legal structures and protection in place from the beginning

Step 6: Hire people who are excellent at what you are not — and pay them fairly

HOW TO PROTECT IT:

Proper business entity from day one — LLC, PLLC, or S-Corp as appropriate

Business insurance: general liability, professional liability, errors & omissions

Operating agreement or partnership agreement in writing — even for trusted partners

Succession plan: what happens to the business if you cannot lead it tomorrow?

Intellectual property protection: trademark your brand, copyright your content

The Debt-to-Freedom Roadmap — How Anyone Can Replicate This

I want to give you, in the clearest terms possible, the sequence that I lived and that this book has built chapter by chapter — so that the path from where you are to where you want to be is not abstract, but traceable. Not a theory, but a map.

The starting point does not matter. I started with an IT background and no nursing credentials, in a new country, with limited financial knowledge, and a generous sister who believed in my potential before I did. The sequence works from any starting point, at any income level, for any healthcare professional willing to apply it with the discipline that clinical training has already instilled.

The Heal Your Wealth Roadmap — From Debt to Generational Freedom

PHASE 1 — FACE THE TRUTH (Chapter 1, 2, 9)

Name the financial reality without performance or shame.

Calculate your net worth — the actual number, not the comfortable estimate.

Identify the inherited money beliefs that are governing your decisions without your consent.

Decision: I am building something different. Starting now.

PHASE 2 — ELIMINATE THE WEIGHT (Chapters 3, 4, 5)

Accept the debt reality and build an elimination plan — Snowball or Avalanche.

Build a baseline budget that functions without overtime.

Give every dollar of extra income a specific destination before it arrives.

Decision: The overtime is a choice, not a necessity. I am building toward that.

PHASE 3 — BUILD THE FLOOR (Chapter 6, 7)

Capture the full employer match in your retirement account — always first.

Open and fund a Roth IRA — tax-free growth for the long horizon.

Buy a home in a neighborhood intentionally chosen for your family's future.

Decision: I am building assets, not just earning income.

PHASE 4 — GROW ABOVE THE FLOOR (Chapter 7, 8)

Add a rental property or REIT to the investment portfolio.

Pursue the certification, the advanced credential, the role that expands your earnings.

Build a secondary income stream from clinical expertise.

Decision: My income is not limited to my primary employer's paycheck.

PHASE 5 — PROTECT WHAT YOU HAVE BUILT (Chapter 10)

Disability insurance with own-occupation definition — in place.

Will, trust, beneficiary designations — current and complete.

Legal entities protecting investment properties and business activities.

Decision: What I built will survive whatever comes next.

PHASE 6 — LEAVE SOMETHING BEHIND (Chapter 11)

Teach your children the financial knowledge you had to find on your own.

Build or support a business that generates value beyond your personal hours.

Mentor one clinician through the financial journey you have completed.

Decision: This does not end with me. It grows from here.

APRNs Can Do This Too

I want to address this directly, because it needs to be said plainly and without qualification: everything described in this book is available to advanced practice registered nurses. All of it.

The real estate. The investment portfolio. The business ownership. The multi-state practice. The executive leadership. The PhD. The pharmaceutical company operates across two countries. The book. The podcast. The financial freedom that allows you to do the clinical work you love without being enslaved to the income it produces.

All of it is available. Not to a hypothetical APRN with more advantages than you have. To you. With your student loans and your rotating shifts and your family obligations and your paycheck-to-paycheck history and your two-hour commute and your children who need you home and your parents abroad who need you solvent. To you, starting from wherever you currently are, with whatever is currently in your account.

The nursing profession has consistently underestimated its financial potential since its inception. We have accepted, as a profession, the narrative that clinical excellence is somehow incompatible with financial ambition — that caring deeply about patients means caring less about building wealth. That is not the truth. It is a story that was convenient for systems that needed our labor and preferred that we not understand our leverage.

I am not angry about that story. I refuse to repeat it.

> ***APRNs can build real estate portfolios. APRNs can run companies. APRNs can retire in financial dignity and leave their children with wealth rather than debt. This is not an aspiration. This is evidence. I am the evidence.***

The APRN who reads this book and applies its principles will not look exactly like me when she finishes. She will look like herself — shaped by her own starting point, her family obligations, her clinical specialty, her entrepreneurial vision, and her definition of financial freedom. That is the point. This is not a template for becoming Caroline Oloo. It is a framework for becoming the fullest, most financially empowered version of yourself. The Caroline version of this story includes Kenya, Texas, East Africa, a pharmaceutical company, and a podcast. Your version will include the specific coordinates of your own extraordinary life. But the principles are the same. The sequence is the same. The outcome — financial freedom, built with intentionality, protected with discipline, and passed forward to the generation watching you — is equally available.

Mentoring the One Behind You

Here is the commitment I want to ask of you as you close this book: find one.

Find one nurse, one NP, one PA, one pharmacist, one therapist who is where you were — deep in the overtime trap, or staring at a credit card statement they do not know how to address, or sitting in a break room performing financial wellness they do not feel, or carrying the weight of two worlds without the financial literacy to manage either of them effectively.

Find that person and have the conversation that someone should have had with you. Not a lecture. A conversation. Share one thing you learned in this book that would have changed something for you if you had known it ten years ago. Recommend a resource. Tell your story honestly — the debt, the second job, the moment you sat down and looked at the numbers and decided something had to change. Give them the map, or at least the first few coordinates.

Financial knowledge is not diminished by sharing. It is amplified. Every clinician who understands how to build wealth and chooses to teach it to another is adding a node to a network of financial literacy that the healthcare profession has been desperately missing. You are not just healing your own wealth. You are healing the financial culture of an entire profession — one honest conversation at a time.

The Ripple a Single Decision Creates

You read this book.

You build the budget, eliminate the debt, buy the home, open the Roth, and start the business.

Your children watch you. They learn not because you told them but because you showed them.

You mentor one colleague. She applies one principle. Her financial trajectory changes.

She tells someone else. That person tells someone else.

You never meet most of the people your decision affected.

You changed their lives anyway.

That is what a legacy looks like from the inside — ordinary decisions, extraordinary reach.

Giving as a Wealth Strategy

Legacy is not complete without generosity. And generosity, properly understood, is not the opposite of wealth-building. It is one of its most powerful expressions.

There is a principle that recurs across cultures, across faiths, across financial traditions: the act of giving — of directing a portion of what you have built toward something beyond your own accumulation — is both ethically essential and practically generative.

Not in a mystical sense. In a structural one. Givers build networks. Givers build reputations. Givers build communities that reciprocate. The person who becomes known in their professional and personal community as someone who gives knowledge, mentorship, and financial support where it is genuinely needed is building social capital that eventually returns in the form of opportunities, partnerships, referrals, and trust.

This does not mean giving indiscriminately or sacrificing your own financial security for others. It means building a giving practice into your financial plan — a percentage of income designated from the beginning, not from what is left over. Ten percent is the number most traditions point toward. Three percent is better than zero. The amount matters less than the habit, and the habit matters less than the intention behind it.

Give to your profession. Give to the community that shaped you. Give to the country you came from, in ways that build capacity rather than dependency. Give to the next generation of healthcare professionals who need the scholarship, the mentorship, and the opportunity that you needed and may or may not have received. Give in ways that carry your values forward — that make the financial legacy you are building about more than your own family's security, as important as that security is.

> ***The most enduring wealth is the kind that was built for more than yourself. Build it wide enough to carry others. That is what transforms a financial plan into a legacy.***

The Life You Are Building Toward

I want to close this book the way it began — with a specific person in a specific moment.

You are retired. Or semi-retired. Or in the season of your career where the work is entirely chosen — every clinical hour, every consulting engagement, every speaking invitation accepted because it aligns with what you care most about, and declined without financial anxiety when it does not.

The mortgage is paid, or the rental income covers it. The children you raised are adults — financially literate adults who understand compound interest, diversification, and the difference between consumer debt and strategic capital, not because of a lecture but because of the model. Your retirement accounts have compounded for decades. Your properties generate monthly income that does not require a single additional shift to sustain. Your business, or the intellectual property you built from your clinical expertise, continues to produce value in your absence.

You wake up, and you do what you love. Not what you must. Not what the budget requires. What you love. The clinical work, the teaching, the writing, the consulting, the mentorship — whatever form the love takes at this season of your life. And you do it without the low-grade financial anxiety that once lived permanently in the background of everything, that followed you through the break room and the shift change and the long drive home from the second hospital.

That anxiety is gone. Not because the world became easier. Because you built something strong enough to hold the life you wanted without requiring that you sacrifice hours of it to sustain the income that funds it. The building took years. The discipline was real. The sacrifice — the downgraded apartment, the debt snowball, the overtime declined for the school pickup, the investment account that stayed invested through every market correction — was real.

And it was worth it. Every single decision.

> ***You did not come this far to arrive at an ordinary life. You came this far to build an extraordinary one—and to hand the map to everyone who comes after you.***

BOARDROOM MOMENT — FINAL

Heal Your Wealth – Chapter 11 Reflection

This is the last Boardroom Moment in this book — and the most important one. Everything that came before it was preparation. This is the declaration.

11. Write your financial legacy statement in full — not as a financial projection but as a declaration. What do you want your financial life to say about you? What do you want your children to inherit beyond assets — what knowledge, what model, what story? Write it in the first person and present tense, as if it is already true: 'My financial legacy is...'
12. Name one person in your professional life who is where you were financially — in the overtime trap, in debt, performing wellness they do not feel. What is one specific thing from this book you will share with them this month? Not as a lecture. As a conversation. Write down what you will say.
13. If you have children or will have children: what is one financial habit or conversation you will introduce into your home this year that did not exist in the household you grew up in? Name it specifically — a savings account they help manage, a conversation about how investing works, the first time they watch you review your net worth.
14. What is the entrepreneurial vision you have been carrying that your financial life is not yet stable enough to pursue on a full scale? Map the distance between where you are now and where you need to be financially to pursue it with genuine capacity. What is the first milestone, and what is your target date to reach it?
15. Return to the legacy statement from the first question of the very first Boardroom Moment in this book — the one that asked you to describe the financial life you are building toward. Read what you wrote then. Now write what you would write today, having completed this journey. Notice what has changed. That change is the beginning of your legacy.

Your legacy is not what you leave behind when you are gone. It is what you build while you are here — and who you build it for. Start today. The generation watching you is already learning.

— — —

A FINAL WORD FROM CAROLINE

To every healthcare professional who reads this book:

I wrote this because someone should have written it sooner.

Because the version of me who arrived in America with ambition and almost no financial literacy deserved a map, and there was not one that spoke to her specifically — to the immigrant nurse, the first-generation professional, the woman managing two worlds while trying to build a third.

So I built the map from within the experience. From the debt and the second job and the overtime trap, and the moment I sat down with every statement on the kitchen table and decided something had to change.

What changed was not my income. What changed was my relationship to it.

That relationship — intentional, honest, courageous, and perpetually curious — is what this book has tried to give you. Not a formula. Not a shortcut. A way of thinking about money that puts you in the driver's seat permanently, regardless of where you are starting from.

You are not behind. You are not too late. You are not too broke or too indebted or too far from the version of this you want for your life.

You are exactly at the beginning of the rest of it.

Now go build something worth leaving behind.

With gratitude and belief in your potential,

Caroline Oloo, MSN, FNP-BC

APRN CAN DO IT, TOO.

And now you have the roadmap.